*This book is dedicated to the memory
of my father, whose support, love, and
encouragement will remain with me always.*

ACKNOWLEDGMENTS

I would like to thank Mark Borke, M.D., emergency medicine specialist in Butte, Montana, and John Bleicher, teacher and education coordinator of Missoula EMS, for their professional wisdom and contributions in the review of the medical material in this book. For those readers who would like to learn as much as they can about the challenging area of emergency wilderness medicine, John's five-day course in Wilderness First Response, given in Missoula, Montana, every winter, is one of the very best anywhere.

Jim Wilson, a dedicated mountaineer and veteran of numerous Alaskan expeditions, among other climbing accomplishments, deserves many thanks for invaluable suggestions offered from a true wilderness expert's point of view.

Special thanks go to Bill Schneider, Falcon publisher, for providing me the opportunity to write this book, and to Russ Schneider, editor and veteran Glacier Wilderness Guide.

Contents

Introduction

For the purpose of this book, wilderness is defined as a remote location more than an hour from professional medical care. For most of us, the concept of wilderness has little to do with the notion of access to medical care and everything to do with the sense that only in wilderness are our spirits truly free. Nevertheless, every time we enter the wilderness we risk injury. We face greater risks to life and limb driving to our backcountry destination, but few of us would venture down the road to the trailhead in our sport utility vehicle without training and experience in the fine art of safe driving, even if the law allowed it. Yet, each year, millions of folks enter wilderness areas with little more than a dab of antibiotic ointment and a prayer.

I have practiced primary care medicine in rural Montana for more than twenty years, yet all of that plus six years as a Boy Scout wasn't enough to drum the point about always being prepared into my head. It took a fairly common injury to my young son to finally drive home the idea. We were at a friend's ranch, near the end of a two-mile walk to a remote section of trout stream. Climbing the last fence before we reached the creek, my son tripped over the top wire, breaking both bones in his wrist as he hit the ground. My truck was back at the house, and the irrigated meadows were undrivable. I did not even have a Band-Aid with me, let alone any useful first-aid equipment. On that long walk back to the ranch, my seven-year-old son bravely cradling his broken wrist in his hand, I promised myself I would never again venture into wilderness unprepared.

USING THIS BOOK

If you seek recreation in the wilderness, common sense dictates you must be prepared for the most common injuries and illnesses you will encounter. Red Cross-approved courses in CPR and basic first aid are a sensible minimum. Further training in wilderness first aid is widely available from other professionals around the country. I also suggest that you read at the very least the first four chapters before going on a trip. This book provides first-aid information and prevention tips for outdoor recreation. It cannot take the place of first aid and CPR classes, but it can refresh your memory prior to a wilderness outing and act as a valuable reference during emergency situations. The basic principle of these courses and the philosophy behind this book is that ordinary people are capable of doing more than they think they can in an emergency. With a little instruction, and a measure of experience, you can acquire the knowledge to successfully cope with a wide variety of emergencies.

PREVENTING ACCIDENTS AND INJURY

The role of proper nutrition, hydration, and clothing in preventing accidents and illness during any wilderness trip cannot be overemphasized. Season after season, wilderness catastrophes can be traced back to the failure of backcountry travelers to eat and drink adequately, and to carry the right clothing and equipment for the conditions they are likely to encounter. Inadequate calorie intake and dehydration can play a role in making conditions such as frostbite, hypothermia, shock, burns, the healing of wounds, infection, illness due to heat, high altitude sickness, diarrhea, and constipation more serious.

Prevention of accident and injury in the wilderness begins long before you leave home. It requires pre-season physical conditioning and sometimes weight loss. A checkup with a doctor makes sense if you are over forty. Always carry rain gear and a first-aid kit. Don't plan more trip than you can handle. Don't climb mountains or crags beyond your abilities without an experienced partner or guide. Take an ice axe and crampons if you plan to cross summer snow, and know how to use them. If you are hiking or climbing in an area prone to rock falls, wear a helmet.

Backcountry adventures can easily increase the body's need for fuel to 4,000 or 5,000 calories a day. Extreme exertion at high altitude can raise that figure even higher. The same is true of water needs. It takes about 2 quarts (liters) of water to maintain a proper state of hydration during a day at the office. The exertion of a wilderness trip can double or triple our daily water requirement, even in winter. This includes water consumed in soups and fruit drinks.

A backcountry diet for trips below 10,000 feet should be more balanced than simple high carbohydrate recommendations of previous years. Try dividing your calories as follows: 40 percent from carbohydrates, 30 percent from protein, and 30 percent from fat. Above 10,000 feet, 70 percent of calories should come from carbohydrates, with the remaining calories evenly divided between protein and fat. Balancing protein, fat, and carbohydrates in this way provides your endurance muscles with a smooth and continuous flow of fuel, and allows for the storage of more calories than can be accomplished with older high-carbohydrate diets alone.

Don't wait until you feel hungry or thirsty to eat or drink; you will always be behind in fuel and fluid balance and will soon exhaust yourself. Prudent drivers don't wait until their car runs out of gas or overheats to fill the tank and radiator. Get into the habit of eating small amounts of nutrient-balanced food and drinking lots of water throughout the day. One of the new balanced energy bars, timetested gorp, bagels, salami, or jerky all work well.

YOU CAN HELP

Realistically, things might happen to you or your companions on a wilderness trip that even a trained medical expert would not be able to treat in the field. Fortunately, these are not the most common injuries and illnesses. With this book and an adequate first-aid kit in your pack, you can do at least some good for almost everyone you encounter who requires first-aid treatment in the backcountry.

One caution, though: the first-aid instructions in this book are intended to help you reach professional medical care safely and comfortably; none of the advice in this book is intended to replace professional medical care whenever it is available. When in doubt, get out or get help!

Appendix A contains a list of items necessary for a basic wilderness first-aid kit. If you wish to expand your knowledge of wilderness medicine, several excellent books on the subject are listed in **Appendix D**.

1

First Response

In the backcountry you can't call 9-1-1. You and your companions are all you have to rely on. This can be frightening, especially if you have never been responsible for the immediate care of a seriously injured or ill person. If you attend first-aid courses, CPR classes, and avalanche awareness seminars, you will feel more confident and be more effective in a wilderness emergency situation. You must immediately decide if the victim is alert or unconscious, if she is breathing, and if her circulatory and nervous systems are functioning normally. Once you have made these critical decisions and acted appropriately, take a few deep breaths. Then move on to your evaluation of less critical conditions.

EVALUATING THE ACCIDENT SCENE

1. Calm and compose yourself and others at the scene. Project a sense of self-confidence, cool-headedness, and compassion.
2. As you approach the scene, try to imagine what might have happened. The way in which a victim is discovered at the scene can help you decide what her injuries are most likely to be. Is she lying at the base of a cliff with her right leg bent at a funny angle, or soaking wet and unconscious on the riverbank, with the litter of a broken canoe scattered around her?
3. Decide if the accident site is safe enough to perform evalu-

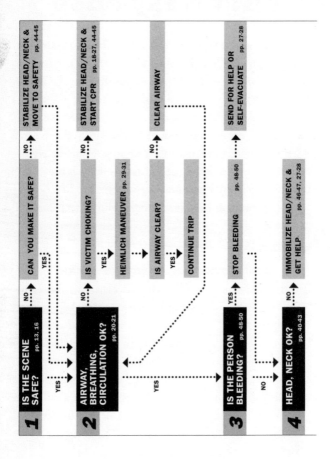

1 IS THE SCENE SAFE? pp. 13, 16

NO ➔ **CAN YOU MAKE IT SAFE?**
- NO ➔ **STABILIZE HEAD/NECK & MOVE TO SAFETY** pp. 44-45
- YES

YES

2 AIRWAY, BREATHING, CIRCULATION OK? pp. 20-21

NO ➔ **IS VICTIM CHOKING?**
- NO ➔ **STABILIZE HEAD/NECK & START CPR** pp. 18-27, 44-45
- YES ➔ **HEIMLICH MANEUVER** pp. 29-31 ➔ **IS AIRWAY CLEAR?**
  - NO ➔ **CLEAR AIRWAY**
  - YES ➔ **CONTINUE TRIP**

YES

3 IS THE PERSON BLEEDING? pp. 48-50

YES ➔ **STOP BLEEDING** pp. 48-50 ➔ **SEND FOR HELP OR SELF-EVACUATE** pp. 27-28

NO

4 HEAD, NECK OK? pp. 40-43

NO ➔ **IMMOBILIZE HEAD/NECK & GET HELP** pp. 46-47, 27-28

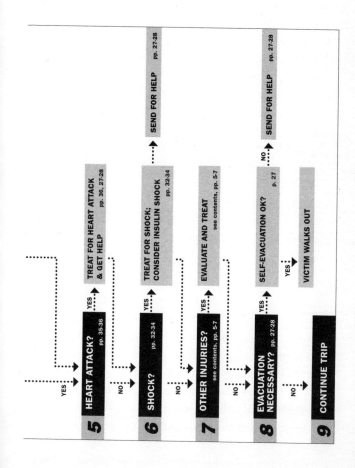

5 HEART ATTACK? pp. 35-36

YES → TREAT FOR HEART ATTACK & GET HELP pp. 36, 27-28

NO ↓

6 SHOCK? pp. 32-34

YES → TREAT FOR SHOCK; CONSIDER INSULIN SHOCK pp. 32-34 → SEND FOR HELP pp. 27-28

NO ↓

7 OTHER INJURIES? see contents, pp. 5-7

YES → EVALUATE AND TREAT see contents, pp. 5-7

NO ↓

8 EVACUATION NECESSARY? pp. 27-28

YES → SELF-EVACUATION OK? p. 27

NO → SEND FOR HELP pp. 27-28

YES → VICTIM WALKS OUT

NO ↓

9 CONTINUE TRIP

ation and treatment. In wilderness, the safety of the rescue party takes precedence over ideal medical management of the victim. Are you or the victim exposed to rockfall, avalanche, fire, or dangerous weather conditions?

4. If the accident site is unsafe, remove the danger or remove the victim. Get out of the rockfall zone or away from the river before you render CPR or first aid. If safety dictates you move the victim before you fully evaluate her injuries, do so only after protecting her spine (see **Spinal Injury,** pages 44-47), if there is any chance she has suffered trauma to the head or neck (fall from height, avalanche, rafting accident).

5. Assess how many victims there are. Treat first those who fail an ABC check (**Airway, Breathing, Circulation**; see pages 20-21), even if others appear to be in great discomfort.

EVALUATING THE VICTIM

1. Ask the victim, "Are you okay?" If she cannot answer, check to see if she is choking or has stopped breathing. Is she clutching her throat and making high-pitched or grunting sounds? If so, treat for **Choking** (pages 29-31).

2. If the victim responds with a coherent answer, then the victim is conscious, breathing, and has a pulse. *You must ask permission from a conscious victim before administering first aid.* The victim has the right to refuse care—disregard this wish only if she appears delirious and self-destructive.

3. If the victim is not choking but is unable to answer, check to see if she is breathing and has a pulse; see the **ABCs**

(pages 20-21). If the victim passes the ABC checklist, CPR is not required. If the victim fails the ABC test, administer **CPR** (pages 18-26).

4. If the victim is breathing and has a pulse, but is not conscious, check for **Head Injury** (pages 40-43) and **Spinal Injury** (pages 44-47).

5. Is the victim bleeding, either inside her clothes or from an obvious wound? Apply pressure with sterile gauze and treat for **Bleeding** (pages 48-50).

6. If she is experiencing shortness of breath, paleness, and squeezing chest pain, treat as if she is having a **Heart Attack** (pages 35-36) and be prepared to administer **CPR** (pages 18-26).

7. If the victim is not bleeding and is not experiencing heart attack symptoms, and she has passed the head injury and spinal injury checklists, evaluate for signs of injuries that do not pose an immediate threat to life (see **Contents,** pages 5-7). Treat injuries or conditions as described in the appropriate chapters.

8. When your evaluation and treatment are finished, decide if the victim requires evacuation from the wilderness and, if she does, can she walk out safely or should someone go for help? If the decision is made to self-evacuate, then continue to monitor the victim for a change in her condition that could require more immediate evacuation. See **Getting Help** (pages 27-28) to decide if evacuation is necessary.

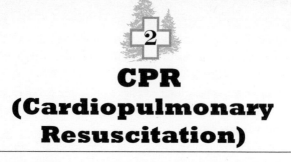

CPR
(Cardiopulmonary Resuscitation)

Cardiopulmonary resuscitation (CPR) is used to revive a person who is not breathing or has no pulse. Cardiopulmonary arrest may occur in the backcountry as a result of massive trauma (a fall from height, avalanche, or lightning strike); an extreme lowering of the body's temperature (hypothermia); near drowning; heart attack; an extreme allergic reaction to plant, reptile, or insect toxins (anaphylaxis); or excessive loss of blood (shock). The most common reason a child may need CPR is that breathing has stopped due to choking, asthma, near drowning, or severe allergic reaction. (See **Choking,** pages 29-30, if you suspect the airway is blocked.)

Successful revival of a person whose heart and lungs have stopped working requires compression of the chest to force blood from the heart, in order to restore circulation, and rescue breathing to supply oxygen to the system. A person who has suffered massive head or chest injuries, or who has had extreme blood loss, cannot be resuscitated in a wilderness setting by CPR alone. A person whose heartbeat is not restored after 30 minutes of CPR is extremely unlikely to survive (exceptions would be someone who has suffered cardiac and respiratory arrest due to severe hypothermia or cold-water near drowning).

The rules for doing CPR in the wilderness are different than they are back in town. In the backcountry, the safety of rescuers and other group members takes precedence over what might be considered standard medical management in an urban setting. Before giving first-aid treatment, make sure you can do so without risk of further injury to the victim, yourself, or your companions. If the victim is in a dangerous location, do not begin treatment until both victim and rescuers are moved to a safe place.

CPR requires professional instruction and regular practice. Consult your local chapter of the American Red Cross or a nearby Search and Rescue Unit. *You cannot learn CPR by reading a first-aid book.* The discussion and diagrams below are intended to refresh your memory if you have not practiced CPR in some time.

If you have reason to believe a person has suffered cardiorespiratory arrest due to trauma, you must stabilize the victim's head and neck before you lift his chin or move his head for your airway check and rescue breathing (see Fig. 1). Logroll the victim onto a sleeping pad or other insulation to keep him off the bare ground. In cold weather, cover the victim with extra clothing or sleeping bags to prevent loss of body heat.

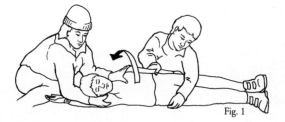

Fig. 1

ABCs (AIRWAY, BREATHING, CIRCULATION)
FOR ADULTS AND CHILDREN

Airway

1. As soon as the victim is in a safe place, check for breathing: watch for chest movement, listen for breath sounds, feel for breath from the nose or mouth. Allow ample time for careful observation.

2. If there are no signs of breathing, or if breathing is weak or shallow, establish an airway with the chin lift maneuver and give two rescue breaths:

    a. keep chin tilted up, but neck straight.

    b. be careful not to force the victim's head back if there is any chance he has suffered a neck injury (see **Spinal Injury**, pages 44-47).

    c. pinch nostrils with thumb and first finger.

    d. cover victim's mouth with your mouth and blow air slowly into his mouth. Pause for several seconds between breaths to allow air to flow out of his chest.

    e. if victim's chest does not rise and fall with rescue breaths, pass two fingers through his mouth to remove any obstructions and clear the airway. If victim does not breathe spontaneously after you have cleared the upper airway, repeat rescue breaths. If chest still does not rise and fall, the lower airway may be obstructed, and you will need to do abdominal thrusts (see Fig. 2):

    • straddle the victim while he lies flat on his back
    • forcibly thrust upward with the heel of your hand at the point on the abdomen below where the breastbone ends.

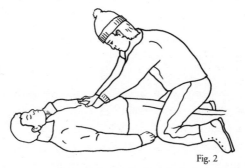

Fig. 2

- pass two fingers through the victim's mouth to remove obstructions.

Breathing

If the victim does not breathe spontaneously after airway is
cleared, resume rescue breathing.

Circulation

Check for a pulse at the carotid artery (see Fig. 3, page 23).
If there is no pulse after 30 seconds, begin chest compressions (start CPR).

   Note: If a child or adult is hypothermic and has no pulse,
and is not breathing, do not attempt chest compressions as
it may cause immediate cardiac arrest. *Hypothermic victims
should receive rescue breathing only.*

ADULT AND CHILD CPR

1. Roll victim onto his back on a firm surface. Move the
   body as a single unit, keeping neck and spine straight if
   he has suffered trauma.
2. Place heel of hand on breastbone in center of chest (about
   2-3 inches below the "V" where breastbone and collar-
   bones meet—see Fig. 4). *Use a CPR Shield if available.*

3. Place your other hand on top of first hand and interlock fingers. Keep shoulders, arms, and hands in a straight line with your weight over them (see Fig. 5).
4. For an adult, compress breastbone about 2 inches with heels of your hands, and repeat 15 times in 10 seconds (80 compressions per minute). For a child, compress the breastbone only 1-1/2 inches 5 times in about 4 seconds, or a rate of 80-100 compressions per minute.
5. Stop chest compression long enough for an assistant rescuer to provide 2 deep mouth-to-mouth breaths after each set of 15 compressions. If performing CPR alone, do 10 chest compressions and give 2 breaths. For a child, stop compressions long enough to provide 1 deep, slow breath after each set of 5 compressions at a rate of 20 breaths per minute.
6. Continue chest compressions and mouth-to-mouth, as above (see Fig. 6).
7. Check for carotid pulse and breathing every few minutes; take about 5 seconds to be sure.
8. If no pulse after 30 minutes, consider stopping CPR if the victim has not been turned over to definitive medical care. (For hypothermic victim, continue to give rescue breathing without chest compressions as noted earlier.)

ABCs (AIRWAY, BREATHING, CIRCULATION) FOR INFANTS

Near drowning, choking, and accidental poisoning are the most common reasons for an infant to require CPR. As is the case with older children, a quick response to a choking infant can save a life. Consult the section on **Choking** (pages

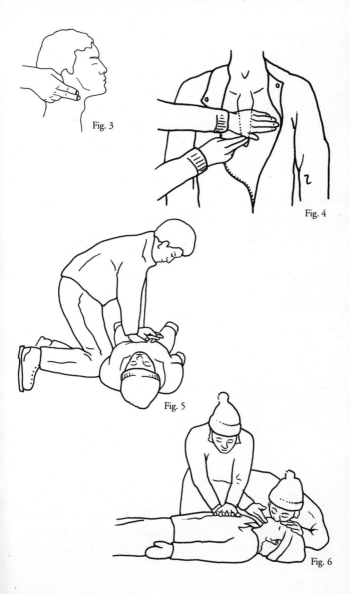

Fig. 3

Fig. 4

Fig. 5

Fig. 6

29-31) if you think the infant stopped breathing because of a foreign object blocking his airway.

If you have reason to believe the infant has suffered cardiorespiratory arrest due to trauma, you must stabilize his head and neck before you lift the chin or move the head for your airway check and rescue breathing. This requires one rescuer to stabilize the head and neck with hands on either side of the infant's head while the infant is moved onto a sleeping pad or other insulation (see Fig. 1, page 19). Cover the infant with extra clothing or sleeping bags to prevent critical loss of body heat.

Airway

1. As soon as the infant is in a safe place, check for breathing: watch for chest movement, listen for breath sounds, feel for breath from the nose or mouth. Allow ample time for careful observation.

2. If there are no signs of breathing, or if breathing is weak or shallow, establish an airway with the chin lift maneuver and give 2 rescue breaths:

   a. keep chin tilted up, but neck straight.

   b. be careful not to force his head back if there is any chance he has suffered a neck injury (see **Spinal Injury**, pages 44-47). If in doubt, follow instructions on immobilization. You will need to do this at the same time you begin rescue breathing and CPR if necessary.

   c. cover infant's nose and mouth with your mouth and blow air slowly into his mouth. Pause for several seconds between breaths to allow air to flow out of his chest.

d. if infant's chest does not rise and fall with rescue breaths, pass two fingers through his mouth to remove any obstructions, and clear the airway. If infant does not breathe spontaneously after you have cleared the upper airway, repeat rescue breaths. If chest still does not rise and fall, the lower airway may be obstructed, and you will need to clear it (see **Infant Choking**, pages 30-31). If the infant's neck has been immobilized because of possible traumatic injury, then perform abdominal thrusts by applying forcible upward pressure with 2 or 3 fingers at the place where the abdomen meets the point of the breastbone.

Breathing

If the infant does not breathe spontaneously after airway is cleared, resume rescue breathing.

Circulation

Check for a pulse at the fold of the arm (see Fig. 7). If there is no pulse after 30 seconds begin chest compressions (start CPR).

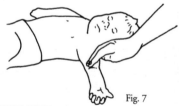

Fig. 7

INFANT CPR

1. Roll infant onto his back on a firm surface, moving the head and body as a single unit.
2. Keep the infant's head tilted back with 1 hand (see Fig. 8a, page 26).
3. Place 2 fingers on breastbone in the middle of his chest (see Fig. 8b, page 26).

4. Compress breastbone 1 inch with your fingers, and repeat 5 times in about 3 seconds (100 compressions per minute) (see Fig. 8c).
5. After each 5 compressions, stop long enough to provide 1 slow (1-1.5 seconds), deep, mouth-to-mouth breath.
6. Continue chest compressions and rescue breathing, as above.
7. Check for carotid pulse and breathing every few minutes; take about 5 seconds to be sure.
8. If no pulse is restored after 30 minutes, consider stopping CPR if the infant has not been turned over to definitive medical care. (If the infant has stopped breathing due to hypothermia, continue rescue breathing as noted above until infant is turned over to definitive medical care.)

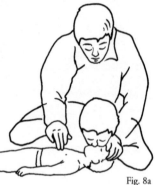

Fig. 8a

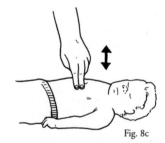

Fig. 8b

Fig. 8c

Getting Help

Knowing which conditions, symptoms, and signs can't be safely treated in the wilderness is crucial. A wise backcountry recreationist knows that few destinations are worth the price of life or limb. Poor judgment on your part may put the lives of rescue professionals or volunteers at risk. You have a moral obligation to evacuate yourself and companions before you have gone past the medical point of no return.

WHEN TO STABILIZE THE VICTIM ON SITE AND GET HELP

If someone is experiencing any of the following:

- Dizzy spells or fainting spells.
- Pulse rate that remains above 110 beats per minute at rest for more than an hour.
- Difficulty catching breath even when at rest.
- Progressive weakness at rest, or with only mild exertion.
- Declining awareness of her surroundings.
- Loss of consciousness for more than 2 minutes, especially after a head injury.
- Pain so severe she simply cannot continue.
- Chest pain that is very clearly not due to an injury to the muscles or bones.

WHEN TO SELF-EVACUATE, IF POSSIBLE

Self-evacuate if any of the following conditions are present:

- Vomiting or diarrhea that gets worse despite basic first-aid treatment.
- Inability to hold down liquids.
- Vomiting blood or bleeding from the rectum.
- An infection that is spreading.
- A psychological state that endangers the person or other members of the group.

Always err on the side of safety—when in doubt, GET OUT or GET HELP!

GETTING OUT SAFELY

Rescues in the wilderness are rarely a matter of brave rangers rappelling from a helicopter—they are most often dirty, sweaty, extremely uncomfortable, and dangerous affairs for everyone, especially the victim. If the injury is severe, and self-evacuation is not an option, send 2 of your party for help, and have 1 or 2 members of the party remain to monitor the injured person for life-threatening changes. If the injury is minor and moving the victim won't make the problem worse, then it is safe to self-evacuate. Whenever possible, those who go for help should not travel alone.

Once out, contact trained emergency rescue personnel: it takes 6 physically fit adults to move an injured person on a litter 100 yards over easy ground, and more than six on difficult terrain. The safety of the rescuers and the injured person's companions takes precedence over what might be considered otherwise ideal medical management.

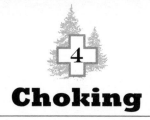

Choking

Choking is a life-threatening emergency wherever it occurs. There is rarely, if ever, enough time to seek professional help. A well-prepared person can easily master the Heimlich maneuver in adults or large children (see below). The procedure for infants is modified but is no more difficult to learn. If you hike or camp in the backcountry with infants or small children, as many parents do, please take the time to learn this simple procedure.

CHOKING IN AN ADULT OR OLDER CHILD

☞ *Signs of Choking in an Adult or Older Child*
- Inability to breathe.
- Cannot speak.
- Hands clutching throat as if strangling.
- High-pitched noises in an attempt to communicate.

✚ *Treating a Choking Adult or Older Child*
1. Ask "Are you choking?" If the choking victim is conscious, he should be able to nod his head.
2. Ask victim's permission to treat with Heimlich maneuver.
3. Stand behind the victim and wrap your arms around him.
4. With your hands interlocked in a fist just below the bottom of the breastbone, squeeze abruptly, forcing air up and out of the obstructed airway (see Fig. 9, page 30). This is the Heimlich maneuver.
5. Repeat maneuver until airway is cleared.

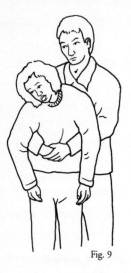
Fig. 9

6. Be prepared to perform CPR if victim loses consciousness.

CHOKING IN AN INFANT

☛ *Signs of Choking in an Infant*

• Coughing that does not stop in a few minutes; may be more forceful than normal.
• High-pitched noises.
• Infant unable to cry in ordinary way.
• Infant unable to breathe.

✚ *Treating a Choking Infant*

1. Hold infant face down, with your hand cradling his chin (see Fig. 10a); use your thigh as a rest.
2. Slap sharply 3 or 4 times between the shoulder blades with the heel of your hand (see Fig. 10b).
3. If no result from slapping, turn infant over, keeping his head lower than his feet, and do 4 or 5 chest thrusts over the center of the breastbone with 2 fingers (see Fig. 10c).
4. Repeat steps 1, 2, and 3 until airway is cleared of obstruction or infant loses consciousness. Be prepared to do CPR if infant loses consciousness.

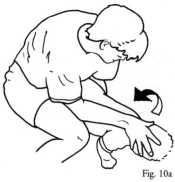

Fig. 10a

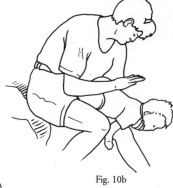

Fig. 10b

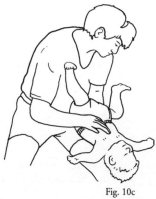

Fig. 10c

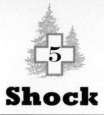

Shock

Shock occurs whenever the flow of blood, with its payload of oxygen and nutrients, falls below the amount required to maintain bodily functions. In the backcountry, shock is seen most commonly as a result of major internal or external blood loss, burns, severe dehydration, severe allergic reactions, insulin reactions in diabetics, or heart attacks. Shock is life threatening, requiring the highest level of rapid evacuation, up to and including helicopter rescue.

☞ *Signs of Shock (All Causes)*
- A catastrophic drop in blood pressure.
- Rapid, shallow breathing.
- A sudden rise in pulse rate, which feels weak, shallow, and "thready."
- Pale, cool, and clammy skin.
- A decline in alertness.

✚ *Treating Shock*
1. Stop all bleeding as quickly as possible (see **Bleeding**, pages 48-49).

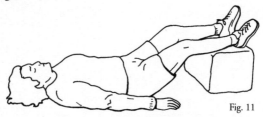

Fig. 11

2. Lay victim down, flat on the ground, with legs elevated (as long as there is no sign of head injury, leg fracture, or spinal injury). See Fig. 11.
3. Keep victim warm with ground pad, blankets, sleeping bags, or extra clothing.

If the victim is alert and thirsty, with no evidence of head injury or abdominal injury (and can swallow without vomiting), she may drink clear fluids, including oral replacement salts in water or sport drink. Fluid intake is adequate when plentiful, clear, colorless urine is produced.

Evacuate all shock victims as soon as possible, using safe procedures. See **Getting Help**, pages 27-28.

For **Severe Allergic Reactions (Anaphylactic Shock)**, see page 101.

INSULIN SHOCK

The dosage of insulin a diabetic routinely uses at home may dangerously lower the blood sugar due to the increased exercise level required for backcountry travel, and can lead to insulin shock. *Insulin shock in the backcountry looks much the same as other forms of shock, and the initial treatment is the same* (see page 34). A person suffering from insulin shock requires a promptly administered dose of a rapidly absorbed carbohydrate (glucose) to bring bodily functions back in balance. If you suspect someone is in insulin shock and follow the steps outlined below, you will cause no harm whether or not they are diabetic, and you may very well save a life.

☞ *Signs of Insulin Shock*
• Suspect insulin shock in an unconscious stranger if signs

of shock are present, and there is no obvious major trauma or blood loss.

- Victims of insulin shock often develop the symptoms slowly and may appear cool, clammy, and drunk, unable to make sense.

✚ *Treating Insulin Shock*

- If you suspect insulin shock, treat the victim for it. If the victim is able to swallow, provide a sweet drink, juice, or candy. If the victim is unable to swallow, sugar or honey smeared inside the mouth will be quickly absorbed. This treatment will not harm a victim in shock for other than diabetic-related reasons. Try two or three tablespoons to start; depending on how low the victim's blood sugar is, you may need to provide three or four tablespoons, or more.

- People with diabetes must recognize their personal insulin shock reactions, and carry their glucose monitoring kit and supplies for appropriate treatment with them. If you are a diabetic, teach your companions how to use your blood sugar monitoring kit, and share your insulin reaction information and supplies of quick-acting glucose with trip companions. Check with your doctor before heading into the backcountry for advice regarding adjusting your insulin dosage, diet, etc.

- If you are the companion of a diabetic, carry backup commercial glucose gel or sugar packets. Smear small quantities of the gel or granules of sugar inside the mouth or under the tongue of a victim in insulin shock; one or two packets of commercial carbohydrate-rich gel will provide 100-200 calories, as would packets of sugar.

6

Chest Pain

Many medical conditions can cause chest pain that mimics the pain of a heart attack. The typical heart attack victim is a middle-aged smoker, but people under thirty can and do have heart attacks. Chest muscle pain, anxiety symptoms, and indigestion or heartburn are the most common causes of chest pain in otherwise healthy adventurers in the wilderness.

HEART ATTACK

A heart attack requires immediate medical attention. Many conditions that are not life threatening can imitate a heart attack, but there is often no way to sort them out in the wilderness. If a person shows any of the signs listed below, alone or in combination, she or he must be considered to be having a heart attack until proven otherwise by professional medical evaluation.

Preventing Heart Attacks

A healthy diet, regular exercise, and consulting a physician before strenuous exercise can reduce the risk of a heart attack on a wilderness adventure. If you are over forty, smoke, or are obese, and have not physically conditioned yourself for the wilderness, a pre-season checkup makes good sense.

☛ *Signs of Heart Attack*
• Pain or pressure in the center of the chest that begins with physical exertion, often described as a crushing or squeezing, unbearable pain.

- Pain that radiates from the chest or upper abdomen up to the neck, jaw, or throat, or down one or both arms.
- Any chest pain accompanied by shortness of breath, sweating (usually on the face and head), nausea, or vomiting.
- Any chest pain accompanied by an overwhelming sense of impending doom.
- Any chest pain accompanied by fainting or lightheadedness.

✤ *Treating Heart Attack*

1. Remain calm and keep the victim as calm as possible.
2. Be prepared to check the ABCs and provide **CPR** (see pages 18-26).
3. Two aspirin will buy time for evacuation by slowing the blood-clotting process. Nitroglycerin tablets used according to a doctor's instructions will buy time for a person with known heart disease.
4. Evacuate ASAP to professional medical attention. Do not attempt self-rescue for a person you suspect is having a heart attack. GET HELP!

SORENESS (MUSCULOSKELETAL CHEST PAIN)

Musculoskeletal chest pain is pain in the muscles and tissues of the chest rather than in the heart or lungs. It is caused by overuse or strain of the muscles and ligaments.

☞ *Signs of Musculoskeletal Chest Pain*
- Aching and soreness due to exercise or injury—carrying a pack, cutting wood, cross-country skiing after a season off, etc.
- Constant, achy tenderness, aggravated by movement of the affected area or finger pressure on the affected area.
- Lasts 2 to 4 days.

✚ *Treating Musculoskeletal Chest Pain*
1. Treat as a muscle strain, with ice and heat (see **RICE**, page 72).
2. Aspirin, acetaminophen, or ibuprofen may be used to relieve pain. Follow instructions on label.

CHEST PAIN DUE TO STRESS

Stress can cause anxiety in anyone at any time. Trips for which you are physically or psychologically unprepared are far more likely to induce stress reactions than those for which you are well prepared. Do not allow your enthusiasm to bully your common sense. Set realistic goals for each trip and remember that getting there is half the fun. Consider wilderness a place to energize the spirit, not inflate the ego.

☞ *Signs of Chest Pain Due to Stress*
- A sense of pressure in the chest or a feeling of suffocation.
- Numbness and tingling of the lips or fingers.
- Trembling.
- Rapid heart rate.
- Rapid, shallow breathing.

✤ *Treating Chest Pain Due to Stress*

1. Stop for rest and a good night's sleep. In the morning, decide whether to continue or retreat.
2. Offer or get reassurance and support of companions.
3. Prescription medications that do not suppress respiration (hydroxyzine, for example) and have no abuse potential may be useful additions to the wilderness first-aid kit. Consult a physician if you are prone to anxiety symptoms. (See **Appendix A** for alternative medications.)

CHEST PAIN DUE TO INDIGESTION

Indigestion is a common complaint in wilderness adventurers. Some meals prepared in the wilderness would upset the digestion of a rhinoceros. Consuming small quantities of nutrient-balanced food and water throughout the day is the sensible way to derive sufficient calories for most endurance activities, and is more efficient than a gargantuan food intake at the end of the day.

Be careful, though—heart attack pain is often confused with indigestion. Heart attack victims can easily talk themselves into a non-heart attack chest pain diagnosis. If there is any doubt as to the origin of the chest pain, or if the pain is not relieved by the simple measures described below, seek immediate professional medical attention.

☛ *Signs of Chest Pain Due to Indigestion*

- Pain experienced after meals and not related to exertion.
- Often made worse by coffee, tea, spicy foods, or alcohol.

✤ *Treating Chest Pain Due to Indigestion*

1. Carry over-the-counter antacid tablets in your first-aid kit; take as directed on the label.
2. Chronic sufferers can purchase Cimetidine over the counter. Follow the instructions on the package. Before you leave for the backcountry, consult your physician to make certain you do not have a medical condition that requires professional care.
3. If no relief in 1-2 hours, assume this to be a condition more serious than indigestion, and arrange for evacuation. If walking or exertion makes the pain worse, assume that you are dealing with a heart attack. Do not attempt self-evacuation. Send someone for help.

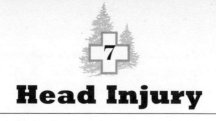

Head Injury

Head injuries are among the most severe wilderness emergencies because they can cause injury to the brain. Head injuries commonly occur during a fall from a height or from a blunt-force blow to the face and neck (as in a snowmobile, kayak, or backcountry ski accident). Serious brain injuries are a primary cause of accidental death. Mountain bikers, snowmobilers, rock climbers, boaters, kayakers, and extreme skiers are at high risk. A great number of these injuries and deaths can be prevented or reduced in severity by wearing a well-fitting helmet appropriate for your sport.

See **Spinal Injury** (pages 44-47) before treating a victim with a head injury, since the two types of injury frequently occur at the same time. If the victim with head injury has lost enough blood to be in shock (see **Shock**, pages 32-34), search for other internal or external injuries. If there are none, the victim's shock is most likely caused by damage to the brain and/or spinal cord.

LOW-RISK HEAD INJURIES

Head injuries in which there is a blow to the head and a loss of consciousness or change in state of alertness for no more than 1 or 2 minutes, and after which the victim is alert, speaking normally, and walking around normally, are considered low-risk head injuries.

👈 *Signs of Low-Risk Head Injury*

- Confusion or loss of memory about the accident that led to the blow for no more than one hour.
- Scalp and facial lacerations which may bleed profusely, but do not penetrate the skull or facial bones.
- "Goose eggs" that swell impressively but are not associated with deformities or depressions of the skull.

✚ *Treating Low-Risk Head Injuries*

1. Stabilize the neck before the victim is evaluated or moved (see Fig. 1, page 19). Once the neck and spine are stabilized, the victim must be logrolled into position for evaluation. Logroll the victim onto a sleeping pad or other insulation to keep her off the bare ground. Her head and neck must remain in line with one another until she passes the spine check (page 45).

2. Apply pressure to the bleeding scalp or face and a cold compress to the "goose egg" (see also **Wounds**, pages 48-50).

3. There is no need to evacuate people with low-risk head injuries because by definition these people are up and walking around under their own power, and in every way appear to be their usual selves within the hour. Nevertheless, these people still require close observation for 24 hours. They should not travel farther into the wilderness during this period of observation. During sleep, awaken the victim every two hours and check for any change in medical condition which would signal that they require immediate evacuation. (See **High-Risk Head Injuries**, below.)

HIGH-RISK HEAD INJURIES

Victims who receive a blow to the face, head, or neck and are unconscious for more than 2 minutes are at high risk for serious brain and/or spinal cord injury. The longer they are unconscious, the greater the risk of more severe brain or spinal cord injury. If any of the signs of severe head injury or skull fracture listed below appear, the victim requires immediate evacuation. High-risk head injury justifies helicopter rescue.

☞ *Signs of High-Risk Head Injuries*

- Unable to wake the person up.
- Changes in level of alertness (difficulty remembering name, location, day of the week).
- Nausea and vomiting that persists or appears worse an hour after the initial blow.
- Headache that gets worse.
- Personality changes.
- Unusual irritability.
- Changes in vision.
- Changes in balance or coordination.
- Slurred speech.
- Convulsive seizures.
- Greatly enlarged pupil on one side and not the other.
- Black and blue marks ("raccoon eyes") surrounding one or both eyes.
- Black and blue marks ("battle sign") behind the ears or on the upper back of the neck.
- Clear or blood-tinged fluid draining from the nose or ears (unless there are cuts, scrapes, or a nasal fracture in the area).

✚ *Treating High-Risk Head Injuries*

1. Immobilize the victim's neck, even if she is alert (see Fig. 12)
2. Once the victim's neck and spine are immobilized, logroll her into position for stabilization, keeping her head and neck in line with one another until you are sure she does not have a spinal injury.
3. Get help ASAP. Do not attempt to self-evacuate the victim (see **Getting Help**, pages 27-28).

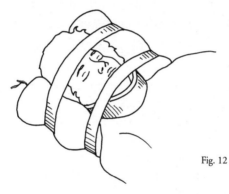

Fig. 12

8

Spinal Injury

The physical forces that can cause a head injury can also cause a fractured neck. People with a low risk head injury can nevertheless have a serious neck and spinal injury. All trauma victims must be thoroughly evaluated for both head and neck injuries. An unstable fracture in the neck can change position, and cause irreversible damage to the spinal cord, which can result in permanent paralysis.

☛ Signs of Head and Neck Injury

The neck (cervical spine) must be stabilized (temporarily made unable to move) in all trauma victims before the victim is evaluated. Ideally, one rescuer should stabilize the victim's neck, while a second carries out the evaluation. Once the neck and spine are stabilized, the victim must be "logrolled" into position for evaluation (see Fig. 1, page 19) so that his head and neck remain in line with one another until you are sure he does not have a spinal injury. Logroll the victim onto a sleeping pad or other insulation to keep him off the bare ground. In cold weather, cover the victim with extra clothing and sleeping bags to prevent loss of body heat. If the victim and rescuers must move to a safe place before the evaluation, then the victim's neck must be immobilized (see **Treating Spinal Injury**, pages 46-47) before he is moved.

☞ *A Trauma Victim's Head and Neck Must Be Immobilized (see Fig. 12, page 43), and the Victim Evacuated Immediately if:*

- He is unconscious, or not fully alert.
- He appears intoxicated.
- He has sustained other injuries that are painful (dislocated joint, fracture of arm or leg, abdominal injury, chest injury), which may mask the pain of a fractured neck.
- There is any complaint of localized, severe pain in the neck.
- He reports pain when you carefully run your finger down his neck from the bottom edge of the skull to the bottom of his neck bone using direct finger pressure.
- He reports numbness, tingling, or loss of sensation anywhere on the extremities, body, or face.
- He cannot wiggle his toes or move his feet, lower and upper legs, hands, fingers, upper and lower arms, or facial muscles.

Note: On rare occasions, trauma victims who "pass" this checklist still turn out to have an unstable fracture of the spine when they reach definitive medical care. The decision to allow a victim to walk out who has "passed" this exam must be made on an individual basis. If the decision is made to immobilize a suspected neck injury in a safe location, while members of the party go for help, and others stay behind with the victim, there can be little criticism of the decision. If the party, and the "passed" victim, decide to walk out of the backcountry and not await professional rescue (assuming no other incapacitating injuries are found), then keep in mind that a fractured vertebra may still be present, and the sudden appearance of any of the checklist items during self-evacuation requires immediate neck immobilization and emergency evacuation.

✤ *Treating Spinal Injury—Immobilization*
(See Fig. 1, page 19, and Fig. 12, page 43)

1. One rescuer temporarily stabilizes the victim's head and neck between his hands and arms.
2. A second rescuer places a neck collar cut from a foam mattress, or a backpack hip belt around the victim's neck, and tapes it to itself to keep it in place. This immobilizes the neck from forward and backward movement.
3. Place rolled-up items of clothing such as jeans, sweaters, or jackets, or two sleeping bags in their stuff sacks, alongside the victim's head and neck to prevent head movement from side to side. These braces or soft splints must be long enough to reach from the level of the collarbone to above the victim's ears.
4. Use duct tape or bandage material to secure the splints by taping them across the forehead and chin so that the head and neck cannot move from side to side. Do not obstruct the airway as you secure your splints.
5. Send for help to evacuate the victim. Maintain immobilization while waiting for, and during, evacuation.
6. Maintain normal fluid intake to prevent hypothermia and shock. Oral fluids, enough to keep the urine clear, are okay if the victim is alert, awake, and not vomiting frequently.

FIRST-AID TIP:
Carry a flexible plastic straw
in your first aid kit to allow
the neck-injured victim to sip
drinks without moving
or choking.

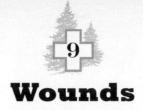

Wounds

BLEEDING WOUNDS

Minor cuts are those without bone, tendon, or joint show-
ing. Bleeding from minor lacerations can be stopped with
simple measures, and does not require evacuation. Major
cuts have more severe bleeding, with exposed bone, tendons,
or joints. These injuries require evacuation because they require skilled surgical repair and prompt medical attention.

✚ *Treating Bleeding Wounds*

1. Wash your hands with soap and water. For your own
   protection (and the victim's), wear clean vinyl gloves to
   treat all bleeding wounds. Wear sunglasses or ski goggles
   if there is a risk of blood splashing into your eye.
2. Stop all bleeding with direct finger or thumb pressure to
   the wound for 15 minutes. Place rolled-up or folded sterile bandage pads or clean items of clothing (T-shirt, socks)
   under your fingers as pressure dressing.
3. If necessary, tie the dressing down with a strip of roller
   gauze or an elastic bandage. Watch for loss of pulse, cool-
   ness of skin, loss of feeling, or severe pain in any extremity
   beyond the pressure dressing. Loosen the dressing immediately if any of these signs or symptoms appear, but
   maintain pressure on the wound with your fingers.
4. When the bleeding has stopped, remove the dressing and
   irrigate all wounds with drinkable water (clear enough
   to drink), or sterile saline if available, using a 30cc sy-

ringe and needle or a large ziplock bag with a small hole in it to deliver the stream of water under pressure. This washes out dirt, debris, and bacteria. Clean the wound and surrounding skin with soap and water. Do not wash the wound with iodine compounds or anything else.

5. Bandage wounds after bleeding has stopped by covering them with a sterile gauze (3- to 4-inch square), wrapping lightly with roller gauze and taping. Antibiotic ointment may be applied to the sterile gauze before placing it over the wound.

6. Close any cuts that will be less painful if closed, such as those over joints, or places where the skin normally folds and creases, or those that are gaping. This will help the person continue the trip or walk out. *DO NOT close wounds with bone, tendon, or joint visible.* The risk of wound infection in closed wounds is significant, and an infected wound can lead to more tissue damage than the original injury.

   To close a bleeding wound safely, gently squeeze the edges of the laceration together and hold them in place with thin strips of adhesive bandage or butterfly bandages (see Fig. 13, page 50). Do not attempt to provide a watertight seal, since some space between the strips will allow for swelling and drainage.

7. If you are more than one day from professional medical care, apply an antibiotic from your first- aid kit following the instructions on the label. All bleeding wounds are at risk for infection. An infection ordinarily takes 1-3 days to become obvious. If you start an antibiotic, continue it for 7-10 days, unless you reach professional

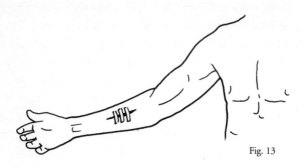

Fig. 13

medical care earlier. You must know about medical allergies before you give anyone (including yourself) an antibiotic. Consult your physician.

8. Change the dressing immediately if it becomes soaked with blood. Otherwise change the bandage daily, but do not remove the adhesive strips unless the wound appears infected (see **Infected Wounds**, pages 53-54).

9. Major lacerations associated with fractures or exposed bone, tendon, or joint should be covered (after bleeding is stopped and the wound irrigated) with sterile bandages of appropriate size, wrapped loosely with flexible gauze, and lightly taped. Such injuries require evacuation. Injuries of this kind in the lower extremities usually do not allow for self-evacuation.

BRUISES

A bruise or contusion is a soft-tissue injury that usually causes bleeding in and under the skin. The bruising may not show up until the day after the injury. Contusions do not break the skin but might accompany a shallow scrape that can bleed quite a bit, or a cut, or, at times, a combination. Blunt trauma from a fall may at first leave no visible mark, but is frequently followed (within minutes or hours) by swelling, pain, and discoloration. Treatment is aimed at reducing swelling, controlling pain, and restoring full function.

✚ *Treating Bruises*

1. Rest the injured part.
2. Apply ice or cold compresses directly to the injured area for 30 minutes every 2 hours. Use a chemical cold pack from your first-aid kit or fill a ziplock bag with snow or cold mountain water. Continue cold application for 48 hours; if pain persists, follow with applications of heat (water of 100-104 degrees F in a plastic sandwich bag) on the same schedule.
3. Compress the swelling with an elastic bandage. If body parts below the compression bandage become cold, painful, or numb, the bandage is too tight.
4. If the injury is on an extremity, elevate the extremity to the level of the heart.
5. Splint for comfort in a position of function (see **Sprains**, pages 71-72). This can be done with a flexible splint, aluminum stays from your pack, or pieces of wood from the forest floor.
6. Watch for and treat signs and symptoms of shock (see **Shock**, page 32).

EMBEDDED OBJECTS

All deeply embedded objects should be left in place—never attempt to remove an embedded object. Doing so could result in severe bleeding, loss of limb, and even death. Use gauze pads placed on either side of the object to keep it from moving, and wrap with gauze rolls just as you would other wounds. Be careful not to move or compress the object further. An object embedded in the eye requires immediate medical attention (see **Object in the Eye**, page 103).

Fish Hooks

DO NOT cut off the hook and try to push it through—this increases both pain and chance of infection. Instead, tie a strong line to the bend in the hook, press down on the eye of the hook, and give the line one hard yank. Pressing down on the eye stretches the wound prior to the removal of the hook. Have someone else do the yanking if you are the one who has been hooked. Never remove a fish hook in the eye (see **Object in the Eye**, pages 105-106).

SCRAPES

Scrapes or abrasions of the surface layers of skin are caused by friction. Mountain bikers call these injuries "road rash." They commonly occur after falls or after being struck by falling rock or tree branches. They can be quite painful and can bleed as much as a cut, although usually more slowly. It is important to care properly for a scrape to reduce the risk of infection.

✚ *Treating Scrapes*

1. Irrigate the wound with water safe enough to drink, or sterile saline if available. Wash away all surface rock, dirt, debris, sand, and loose tissue.
2. Clean vigorously with soap and water. Scrub the surface of the wound with a sterile bandage so that all visible foreign matter is removed. This usually is quite painful. If you have an anesthetic ointment, apply it directly to the skin surface and wait 5-10 minutes for the anesthetic to work before scrubbing.
3. Apply a light coat of antibiotic ointment.
4. Apply sterile bandage of appropriate size and wrap with roller bandage (or elastic bandage if the swelling is severe).
5. Change sterile bandage every day for first 2-3 days.

INFECTED WOUNDS

Despite your best efforts, some wounds will get infected. An infected wound shows redness for more than 1/4 inch along the margins of the wound along with swelling, increasing pain, and possible drainage of pus. It usually takes several days to a week after the injury for an infection to become noticeable.

✚ *Treating Infected Wounds*

1. Remove the bandage and open the wound edges by gently pulling them apart. If there is an infection the wound edges will separate easily and painlessly.
2. Irrigate the wound with water safe enough to drink; wash away all pus and tissue debris without using pressure. DO NOT use a syringe and needle to increase pressure

in this case. You don't want infected material forced back into the tissue.

3. Apply antibiotic cream lightly.

4. Re-bandage the wound with sterile bandages, leaving the wound edges apart to allow it to drain.

5. Change the bandage as often as it becomes soiled with blood or pus that soaks through; otherwise change the bandage daily.

6. If you have not done so before, start an oral antibiotic (Cephalexin is a good choice) from your first-aid kit, following instructions on the label. You must be aware of medical allergies before you give anyone (including yourself) an antibiotic. Consult your physician.

If the infection shows signs of clearing up (no fever or chills; no redness or swelling; pain getting better) over 1 or 2 days' time, you can likely continue the trip, but finish a full 10-day course of the antibiotic, or as instructed on the label. If you are not certain things are definitely better 1 or 2 days after you begin treatment, evacuate and seek professional medical attention.

10

Blisters

Blisters have probably ruined more backcountry trips than anyone can count. A minor annoyance at home, they are potentially crippling in the backcountry if not properly cared for. Prevention of blisters is relatively simple and superior to the best treatment.

Preventing Blisters

Make sure new boots or hiking shoes fit with the sock combination you will wear in the backcountry. A good-fitting boot fits snugly over the arch, but not tightly, and does not permit heel rise when walking up or down an incline. You should have about 1/2 inch of space between the toes and the front of the boot. This will prevent damage to your toes and toenails on steep downhill trails.

Your regular shoe size is only a rough guide to what size boot will fit. No two manufacturers size their boots exactly the same way. Heel lift of more than 1/8 inch or pain anywhere during fitting will only get worse with time. Choose a different boot.

Break in boots on short hikes (10 to 15 minutes a day to start, gradually progressing to 45 minutes to 1 hour), 3 or 4 times a week with a pack on. Do this long before your first backcountry excursion. There is no such thing as too much break-in time, and the break-in can also serve to physically condition you for your trip.

On the trail, cool a "hot spot"—a painful red area that warns of blisters to come—as soon as you become aware of it. Soak your feet in cold water or expose them to the air until the hot spot cools down, and change your socks for a dry pair. Bandage persistent hot spots with molefoam and duct tape. If you know where your usual hot spots are, tape them before you start your break-in period. To prevent infection, clean the area with soap and water before bandaging. Wear dry socks every day, and use foot powder to keep your feet dry.

✚ *Treating Blisters*

1. Clean the skin around and over the blister with mild soap. Pat dry.
2. Lightly paint the entire blister with iodine pads or solution from your first-aid kit.
3. Make a small cut with your scissors (wipe them with iodine first) in the dead skin at the bottom of the blister. This top layer of skin has already been separated from its nerve supply, so opening it should not cause pain.
4. Cover the blister area with a sterile, transparent, air- and moisture-permeable dressing; Tegaderm works well. If the area under the broken blister looks like a shallow crater or is oozing fluid or blood, cover it with a sterile hydrocolloid dressing, such as Duoderm. Blister dressings maintain a moist wound environment to promote healing, and they reduce pain.
5. Place molefoam over the dressing to pad it, and tape in place.

Lightning Injury

Lightning kills more people in the United States than any other natural force—about 300 people each year. Many of those killed are backcountry travelers. On a happier note, only 20 to 30 percent of lightning strikes are fatal. Statistically, only those victims who suffer immediate cardiopulmonary arrest will die (unless they receive CPR, which is not always successful); the remainder of victims may suffer a variety of injuries, some severe, but they will survive.

It is not true that a victim of lightning strike remains "charged" and therefore a danger to her rescuers. DO NOT delay CPR in a lightning strike victim because of a fear that she will electrocute you.

Avoiding Lightning Strikes

Start treks and climbs in early morning during thunderstorm season. Plan to be back at camp or on unexposed ground by one or two o'clock in the afternoon. Be aware of weather forecasts, and be prepared to seek shelter wherever possible.

During a thunderstorm, put down fishing rods, ice axes, trekking poles made of metal, or other objects with metallic components. Take off crampons. Avoid the highest and the lowest ground. Do not seek shelter under isolated tall trees—instead, go into thick, uniform groups of trees, brush, or boulders. If you are near a cave, seek shelter there only if it is dry. If you are boating or swimming, get to shore. If you are at a trailhead, stay inside your vehicle.

Spread your group out if caught in the open, staying 10 to 20 feet apart. Maintain visual contact. Squat or crouch with your feet close together; a foam mattress or climbing rope under your feet will provide some insulation from the ground.

✠ *Treating Someone Struck by Lightning*

Remember your ABCs—Airway, Breathing, and Circulation (see pages 20-21). And assume, for safety's sake, the victim has a neck injury until proven otherwise.

1. Stabilize the unconscious victim's head and neck before you lift the chin or move the head for your airway check and rescue breathing (see pages 44-46).

2. With the neck and spine stabilized, logroll the victim onto a sleeping pad or other insulation to keep his body off the bare ground (see Fig. 1, page 19). In wet or cold weather, cover the victim with extra clothing or sleeping bags to prevent loss of body heat.

3. Initiate CPR immediately to a breathless, pulse-less victim (see **CPR**, pages 18-25). If the victim's heartbeat is restored, he may remain unable to breathe on his own. If this happens, continue rescue breathing during evacuation.

If there are multiple victims, treat the unconscious first, because those who are conscious are already recovering (they may have other injuries, however), but those who require CPR must be resuscitated. Victims whose pulse and heartbeat do not return within 30 to 40 minutes are unlikely to survive.

Survivors of lightning strike should be evacuated to definitive medical care after fractures are splinted, bleeding is controlled, and the spine immobilized (see pages 46-47).

Illness Caused by Heat

Heat edema (swelling of the hands and feet) and *heat syncope* (fainting, with quick recovery) are common among unacclimatized travelers in hot and humid backcountry. They are not medically serious and are self-correcting, but serve as a warning to slow down, cool off, and increase fluid intake. On the other hand, *heat cramps, heat exhaustion,* and *heat stroke* are progressively severe medical conditions caused by the body's failure to adapt to hot weather. Recognition and treatment of heat cramps and heat exhaustion reduce the risk of heat stroke, a potentially fatal illness.

Obesity, poor physical conditioning, thyroid disease, diabetes, heart disease, lack of sleep, and fatigue increase your susceptibility to heat illness. Antihistamines, cold preparations, and beta-blocker blood pressure medications can interfere with sweating; if you regularly take any of these medications, consult your physician before a hot weather backcountry trip. Infants and children are at greater risk for heat-related illness because they are less able to acclimatize to a hot environment. As in most illnesses we might experience during wilderness travel, prevention is a whole lot easier than cure.

Preventing Heat-Related Illness
1. The *most critical* preventive measure is increased water

intake. Don't wait until you are thirsty to replace fluids. Drink a pint (500 ml) of cool, flavored water or sport drink diluted to half strength before the start of physical activities. Drink a glassful (250 ml) every 20 to 30 minutes while exerting yourself in unaccustomed heat. It's easier and more useful to pack the weight of water inside your body than inside your pack. Drink frequently.

2. Maintain a pale, clear urine. Closely monitor the fluid intake of children during summer outings. Have them drink a half-glass of cold, flavored water once or twice every hour during hot weather activities, even if they are not thirsty. Monitor the frequency and color of urine. Clear urine every hour or two is the goal.

3. Balanced oral replacement salts are the safest way to replace electrolyte loss during heat stress. Carry a few packages with you on trips to hot, humid climates. Avoid using salt tablets for salt replacement; they irritate the stomach and slow the entry of critical fluids into circulation.

4. Wear lightweight, light-colored, loose-fitting clothing. Lightweight cotton clothing is a good choice in hot, dry weather because it holds moisture and cools you as the moisture evaporates. In humid climates, lightweight, porous synthetics are a better choice. Avoid the windproof or waterproof versions.

5. Avoid strenuous exertion during hot, humid weather to which you are not accustomed. Start a strenuous trip at first light (or earlier) and rest in the shade during the hottest part of the day. Wait until the temperature drops late in the day to resume trekking.

6. Avoid using alcohol and drugs. Alcohol lowers the body's innate ability to respond to heat stress. The most commonly abused street drugs tend to speed up the rate at which your body produces heat.

HEAT CRAMPS

Heat cramps are severe muscle cramping which begins after strenuous exercise during hot weather. Heat cramps can also be caused by consuming water with inadequate sodium replacement.

✠ *Treating Heat Cramps*

1. Replace lost fluids with cool water (can be flavored) to which is added 1/4 teaspoon of table salt per quart (liter), or a package of balanced oral replacement solution.
2. Rest in a cool, shady spot. Resume activities when cramps are gone; gentle massage helps. If cramps return, take a rest day.

HEAT EXHAUSTION

A more severe imbalance in the body's water and salt balance, along with an abnormal elevation of temperature (up to 104 degrees F), produces a more serious condition known as heat exhaustion. If you only drink when you feel thirsty, you will fall farther and farther behind in your fluid and electrolyte requirements. Untreated heat exhaustion can progress to heat stroke, a medical emergency.

You do not need a thermometer to treat heat exhaustion or heat stroke, but if you have one, so much the better. Disposable oral thermometers are available from many surgical supply distributors. They can provide a rough estimate of core temperature, which is usually about 1 degree higher than oral readings.

☞ *Signs of Heat Exhaustion*

- Feelings of weakness, extreme fatigue, loss of appetite.
- Headaches, dizziness, sweating, rapid pulse.
- Nausea or vomiting.
- Muscle cramps.
- Skin is pale, cool, and moist ("clammy").

✚ *Treating Heat Exhaustion*

1. Stop physical activities.
2. Remove victim to shade; lay the victim down with feet elevated to 30-degree angle.
3. Replace salt and water loss with cool oral rehydration solution or lightly salted water (1/4 teaspoon per quart) by mouth, at the rate of one-half glass every 10-15 minutes until the symptoms improve and the victim is able to produce pale to clear urine.
4. Remove hot, sweat-soaked clothing, wet the skin with cool water, and fan the victim to hasten cooling.

Recovery may take 24 hours. To monitor progress in heat exhaustion or heat stroke, pay close attention to the victim's improvement (or lack of improvement) in his state of alertness, level of comfort, and urine output. Fluid balance is restored when the urine is pale or colorless, and is passed two or three or more times a day. If you have a thermometer, check temperature every hour or so until it starts to drop below your first reading. If the temperature rises, increase fluid therapy until it begins to drop.

HEAT STROKE

There is not always a clear line between heat exhaustion and early-stage heat stroke. The temperature of heat stroke victims is higher than that of heat exhaustion cases (more than 105 degrees F), and heat stroke victims are less alert, more confused, and irrational. The presence of central nervous system symptoms in a heat-stressed victim is sufficient to make the field diagnosis of heat stroke.

Left untreated, heat stroke victims lapse into coma and suffer cardiac arrest. Heat stroke comes on more quickly in high-risk individuals such as children, infants, overweight people, and the elderly, or people with heart disease, diabetes, thyroid disease, or cardiovascular disease.

☞ *Signs of Heat Stroke*
- Extreme agitation, confusion, hallucinations, drowsiness, disorientation, loss of balance, or coma.
- Skin hot, dry, and red in classic cases, but some healthy young victims continue to sweat and have cool, pale skin.

✚ *Treating Heat Stroke*
Heat stroke is life threatening. Remember your ABCs (see pages 20-21) if you are treating an unconscious victim. Start CPR if needed.

1. Cool victim as quickly as you can. Place victim in shade; lay him down with feet elevated. Remove hot, sweat-soaked clothing. Immerse victim in cold water if possible, or place ziplock bags full of cold water, items of clothing soaked in cold water, or ice alongside neck, armpits, and groin, and fan the victim.

2. Do not give oral replacement fluids until victim is cooled down (temperature below 104 degrees F), awake, alert, and can drink without vomiting.

3. Pay close attention to the victim's improvement in his state of alertness, level of comfort, ability to tolerate oral fluids, and increased urine output.

4. If you have a thermometer, check temperature every hour until it starts to drop below your first reading. If the temperature rises, increase external cooling until it begins to drop. When temperature drops below 102 degrees F, slow down external cooling efforts, continue oral fluids (if victim is alert enough to drink), and continue to monitor the victim.

5. Evacuate as soon as possible.

13

Burn Injury

Burns are fairly common in the backcountry. Campfires get out of control, cookstoves flare up inside tents, and hikers get trapped in wildfires. Burns are classified according to the depth to which they penetrate the skin and the total amount of surface area that is burned.

First-degree burns injure only the superficial layer of skin, which is reddish or pale and painful, but without blister formation. Sunburn is a first-degree burn.

Second-degree burns are partial thickness burns that blister.

Third-degree burns are full-thickness burns, which penetrate all the skin layers and may burn underlying tissue as well. The skin is pale or charred, and there is no blistering, although surrounding areas may have blistering burns in addition. Skin usually has no sensation of pain because the sensory nerves have been burned.

When To Evacuate a Burn Victim

The following conditions require management with intravenous fluids and, often, surgical care. Evacuate burned victims with the following signs as rapidly as possible:

- Blistering burns covering more than 5 percent of body surface.
- Any blistering burn of critical areas: face, eyes, ears, hands, feet, or genitals.

THE RULE OF NINES AND ONES

Use this rough guide to estimate the percent of total body surface area covered by burns:

Each palm = 1% body surface area.

Each arm = 9% body surface area (total front and back).

Each leg = 18% body surface area (total front and back).

Torso = 36% body surface area (18% front, 18% back).

Head and neck = 9% body surface area (total front and back).

Genitalia = 1% body surface area.

- All full-thickness burns. Full-thickness burns of more than 10 percent of body surface require rapid evacuation; full-thickness burns of less than 10 percent of body surface will require professional medical attention within 2-3 days, but rapid evacuation is not necessary if the person is able to tolerate oral fluids and is able to walk out.
- Burns accompanied by any additional serious trauma (injury to head, spine, chest, or abdomen; fracture of pelvis or long bone of leg or ankle).

Note: First-degree burns (including sunburn) do not require evacuation unless they cover more than 20 percent of the body surface and are accompanied by fever, chills, nausea, or vomiting.

✠ *General Treatment of Burns*

1. As quickly as possible—within seconds if you are able—remove the heat source or smother flames with a blanket.
2. Remove jewelry and clothing from the burned area, but do not pull off items stuck to the skin.
3. Irrigate the burned area with the cleanest cold water you have to remove all dirt and debris; if the burn is greater than 20 percent of total body surface area, watch for hypothermia. DO NOT apply ice to a burn wound. It will increase the severity of the injury.
4. Elevate a burned extremity to reduce swelling. Cover serious burn wounds with bandages as described below.
5. Stabilize the victim's body temperature. The loss of skin causes loss of body heat in burns greater than 20 percent of body surface.

FIRST-AID TIP:

Travel on snow or glacier ice, even on cloudy days, requires full eye protection to prevent injury. Wear side-shield sunglasses or goggles (100 percent UV reduction, 90+ percent visible light reduction) and use sunscreen of the highest protection level.

---

6. Encourage the victim to drink as much fluid as she can tolerate as long as she is not vomiting. Rehydrate with cool or cold water. Add 1/4 teaspoon salt to each quart (liter) of water, or carry commercially available rehydration salts.

7. Maintain an hourly flow of pale, clear urine for the first 24 hours.

✤ *Treating First-Degree Burns and Sunburn*

1. Gently wash the burned area with soap and lukewarm water. Pat dry.

2. Treat pain with ibuprofen as necessary. (See **Appendix A** for alternative medication suggestions.) Over-the-counter gels containing aloe vera can reduce the pain of a first-degree burn. Cool compresses will reduce the pain of first-degree burns and sunburn.

✤ *Treating Second-Degree Burns*

1. Clean the burned area as above. Do not open intact blisters unless on palms of hands or soles of feet. If blisters break, remove the dead skin with a scissors and forceps (sterilize these by boiling); wear clean or sterile gloves.

2. Apply a light coating of antibiotic cream. (See **Appendix A** for suggestions.)

3. Cover the burned area with a non-stick bandage or a water-retaining colloidal burn dressing such as Spenco Second Skin. Wrap snugly but not tightly with roller gauze. Tape in place.

4. Splint burns of the hand in a position of natural function (see Fig. 14). Place a roll of sterile gauze in the palm,

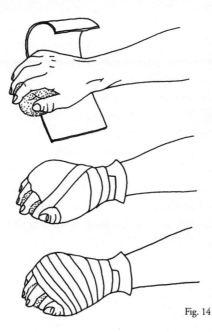

Fig. 14

then wrap the fingers and hand in the position the hand takes naturally when holding a ball.

5. Treat for pain with aspirin. (See **Appendix A** for alternative suggestions.)

6. Change the bandage every day. If you notice signs of infection (fever, foul-smelling drainage, pus, swelling or redness, pain in areas of skin next to the burn), open the blister and irrigate with clean water. Redress, then evacuate for professional medical care.

✚ *Treating Third-Degree Burns*

Remember the ABCs—check the airway, and for breathing, check the circulation; begin rescue breathing and CPR if necessary (see pages 18-26).

1. Clean and irrigate as above.
2. Apply water-retaining colloidal burn dressing, such as Spenco Second Skin.
3. Treat adjacent areas of skin with lesser-degree burned tissue.
4. Manage pain with ibuprofen as directed on the label. (See **Appendix A** for alternative suggestions.)
5. Evacuate to definitive medical care (see **Getting Help**, pages 27-28).

Bone and Joint Injuries

Strains and sprains are stretching and tearing injuries to ligaments and tendons. Along with broken bones (fractures), they are among the most common back-country injuries. You can tell when a fracture has dislocated the parts of the bone that are broken because the injured limb looks deformed. Sometimes you can hear or feel the ends of a broken bone grating against one another. Unfortunately, not all fractures result in obvious dislocation and deformity or grating bone ends. For this reason, the initial field treatment of most sprains, strains, and fractures is similar.

STRAINS AND SPRAINS

Strains and sprains are often the result of a fall. Symptoms are similar to those of a fracture, particularly in the ankle. If you have any doubt, treat the injury and remain in camp for 1-2 days to see if pain, swelling, and inability to move the injured part improve. If they do, it is safe for the person to walk out. If not, assume there is a fracture and arrange for evacuation.

☛ Signs of a Strain or Sprain
- Tenderness to the touch.
- Discoloration ("black and blue").
- Swelling in a joint or muscle.
- Pain with movement of the injured part.

✚ *Treating Strains and Sprains*

1. A helpful memory device to recall the steps of treatment is known as **RICE:**
   - **R**est the injured part for 48-72 hours.
   - **I**ce the swelling (use a plastic bag with ice, snow, or cold creek water). Apply cold for 20 minutes every hour, placing a towel or clean item of clothing next to the skin. Continue for 48-72 hours.
   - **C**ompress the swelling with an elastic bandage and immobilize the sprained joint.
   - **E**levate the injured part to lessen swelling and pain.
2. Treat pain with aspirin, acetaminophen, or ibuprofen.

Wrapping an Ankle

In the ankle, the most commonly sprained joint, compression and splinting are accomplished with an elastic bandage by wrapping it in a cross-woven pattern (see Figs. 15a-d, page 73). Don't remove the victim's boot unless he does not have feeling in the toes; instead, simply wrap the bandage over the boot. If possible, a 2-day trip delay to allow the swelling to go down is preferable.

BROKEN BONES

Oftentimes even a trained professional can't diagnose a broken bone without an X-ray. For first aid in the wilderness, adhere to the basic rules of splinting, immobilization, and evacuation. If displaced and dislocated fractures immediately threaten the nerve and blood supply of an extremity, the loss of blood supply below the fracture site can lead to the loss of the limb. These grossly displaced fractures must be straightened quickly if the limb is to be saved (see page 76).

All fractures require evacuation and medical attention. Fractures or suspected fractures of the pelvis, hip, thigh, knee, or lower leg (tibia) require rapid evacuation to definitive treatment. Monitor for shock (see **Shock**, page 32).

Simple (closed) fractures are those without a break in the skin. Open fractures are fractures with any break in the skin over the fracture, up to and including those from which the ends of a bone protrude. This differentiation is important because of differences in treatment.

If an ankle injury that might be a fracture is immobilized and elevated, and there are no additional injuries that require immediate evacuation, it is okay to wait two or three days to see if the pain and swelling improve enough to walk out.

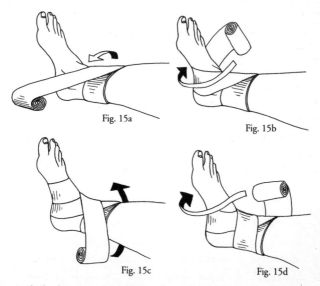

Fig. 15a

Fig. 15b

Fig. 15c

Fig. 15d

In the backcountry, the ankle may be wrapped with the hiking boot on.

Victims with fractures of the upper extremity that are immobilized can walk out if there are no other serious injuries.

An adequately prepared individual must learn a great deal more about the treatment of fractures and dislocations than could be included here. Advanced splinting and immobilization techniques require professional training and practice.

☛ *Signs of a Simple (Closed) Fracture*

- Pain and tenderness over the fracture site.
- Swelling and discoloration due to bleeding under the skin.
- Obvious deformity or severe angulation of the limb.
- The sound of bone ends grating under the skin.
- Victim can not bear weight on injured lower extremity.
- No evidence of break in skin or protruding bone ends.

✚ *Treating a Simple Fracture*

1. Immobilize all fractures or suspected fractures by splinting (see below). Carry a commercial flexible splint in your first-aid kit or improvise with sticks, foam pads, aluminum pack stays, ski poles, skis, folded maps, or rolled items of clothing and adhesive tape. DO NOT attempt to straighten a closed fracture unless it is cutting off the blood or nerve supply to the extremity, signified by numbness, tingling, extreme pain, and/or bluish color below the fracture site. Otherwise, splint it in the position in which you find it. If a fracture requires straightening to prevent a loss of circulation in the limb, do it as soon as possible after the injury (see pages 76-80).

2. Treat swelling with ice or cold water in plastic pouches, as for a sprain.

3. Treat pain with ibuprofen according to directions on the label. (See **Appendix A** for alternative suggestions.)

☞ *Signs of an Open Fracture*

- Broken skin or visible bone ends.
- Pain and tenderness over the fracture site.
- Swelling and discoloration due to bleeding under the skin.
- Obvious deformity or severe angle of the limb.
- The sound of bone ends grating under the skin.
- Victim cannot bear weight on injured lower extremity.

✚ *Treating an Open Fracture*

1. Irrigate the wound with water that has been made safe enough to drink until all dirt and debris are washed away. Do not close the wound with adhesive strips, staples, sutures, or glue—instead, cover it with several bandages and tape to hold in place.

2. DO NOT attempt to straighten an open fracture unless it is cutting off the blood or nerve supply to the extremity (numbness, tingling, pain, bluish color). Otherwise splint it in the position in which you find it. If an open fracture requires straightening to restore the blood supply or allow splinting, do it as soon as possible after the injury (see below).

3. Evacuate all open fractures as quickly as conditions allow. If evacuation is delayed more than 3 hours, you can administer an oral antibiotic if you have one with you. (See **Appendix A** for suggestions.)

STRAIGHTENING AND SPLINTING

✚ *Straightening a Deformed Fracture*

Only those deformed fractures that are cutting off the blood supply to an extremity should be manipulated in the field— this kind of fracture most commonly occurs in the leg, ankle, or elbow. Before you attempt fracture manipulation to save a limb that is having blood supply cut off, tell the victim what you propose to do and why, and what the risks are. The main risk is more damage to the blood supply, and more bleeding into the muscles surrounding the bone. An attempt to straighten a fracture can also fail to restore blood supply because the fractured bone ends have already cut the arterial supply. *You must have the injured person's agreement and understanding before you attempt fracture manipulation.*

1. One person holds the limb above the fracture site to provide an anchor for the traction. Most commonly this will be a fracture of the leg between the knee and the ankle, or the ankle, or the elbow. The person providing the anchor for the traction must not allow movement of his anchor.

2. A second person holds the extremity below the fracture site and straightens the deformity with a gentle, steady, straight pull. Use the opposite, uninjured limb as a guide. The object is to restore circulation, not to provide definitive care for the fracture. Straightening the fractured bone as best you can will relieve pressure on the blood supply. If the foot or arm turns pink, warms up, and the pain is reduced, you have accomplished your goal.

3. When the fracture is straightened and circulation restored, splint to immobilize.

❖ *Splinting the Hand or Fingers*

1. Bandage the hand in a natural position with a sock or a roll of gauze in the palm (see Fig. 14, page 69).
2. A forearm sling is necessary to keep the hand and fingers elevated. Use a commercial triangular bandage or improvise a sling using the victim's shirt and safety pins (see Fig. 16, page 78).

❖ *Splinting the Wrist or Forearm*

1. Pad the elbow with foam from a packframe or sleeping pad or items of clothing.
2. Splint from just above elbow to palm of hand with commercial flexible splint, aluminum pack stays, pillows, or sticks. Wrap with elastic bandage or tape.
3. A forearm sling with an upper arm binder is necessary to keep the hand and fingers elevated and the fracture immobilized. Use a commercial triangular bandage or improvise a sling using the victim's shirt, safety pins, and an item of clothing (see Fig. 16, page 78).

❖ *Splinting the Elbow, Upper Arm, or Shoulder*

1. Pad the elbow with foam from a packframe or sleeping pad or items of clothing.
2. A forearm sling with an upper arm binder is necessary to keep the hand and fingers elevated and the fracture immobilized. Use a commercial triangular bandage or improvise a sling using the victim's shirt, safety pins, and an item of clothing for the binder (see Fig. 16, page 78).
3. If the fingers or hand become cool, blue, or painful, loosen the binder.

✚ *Splinting the Collarbone*

A fracture of the collarbone can be felt by running a finger over the bone. The person will report pain at the fracture site when you do this.

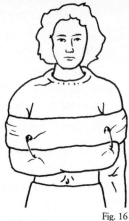

1. Pad under the arms to protect the nerve and blood supply.
2. Wrap an elastic bandage in a figure eight, over the clothing, as shown in Figs. 17a-b.

Fig. 16

✚ *Splinting a Fractured Thigh Bone*

Fractured thigh bones can cause massive internal bleeding if they are not splinted in a position of traction. For this reason, all fractured thigh bones should be splinted before evacuation. Traction is a continuous pulling force, applied temporarily by a rescuer, or longer by means of a splint. Contraction of the thigh muscles, as a reflex response to the fracture, without traction, causes severe pain. Traction makes the victim safer and far more comfortable. The splint shown in Fig. 18, page 80, and described below will provide comfort and help control bleeding around the fracture, but it is not sufficient for extended transport out of the wilderness. This injury justifies the use of helicopter evacuation.

1. One member of the party should promptly apply a gentle, straight pull (traction) from the ankle, on the ground, after the victim is evaluated. A straight pull with continuous steady force is maintained while a second member of the party prepares the splint.

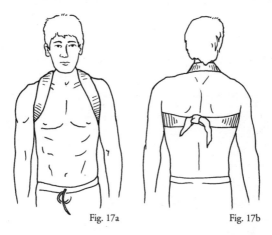

Fig. 17a   Fig. 17b

2. Wrap an elastic bandage over the fracture site to control bleeding. DO NOT remove victim's shoe or boot.
3. Pad the ankle with a foam mattress cut to size, a pillow, or a jacket, and tape. Do the same around the top of the thigh where it joins the buttock.
4. Fashion a traction device (see Fig. 18, page 80) with ski poles, sticks, or ice axe, and bandage material—duct tape works best.
5. Roll an item of clothing under the knee to flex the knee at a 5- or 10-degree position and wrap it in place with padding and tape to protect the side of the knee where the splint will be taped. A flexed knee is more comfortable during evacuation.
6. Maintain a straight, steady pull from the ankle (traction) as the splint is taped into position on the thigh and ankle padding.

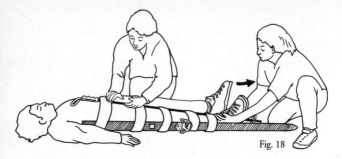

Fig. 18

7. If the foot or toes become cool, numb, or painful, loosen the ankle padding and rewrap.
8. Get help for evacuation. See pages 27-28.

✠ *Splinting an Ankle, Lower Leg, or Knee*

1. Roll a foam pad or partially inflated air mattress and place it under the foot like a stirrup on a saddle (see Figs. 19a-b).
2. Wrap the padding with an elastic bandage or roller gauze and tape it in place.
3. Splints for the lower leg or knee must extend above the knee.
4. If the toe or foot becomes cool, blue, or painful, loosen the bandage.

✠ *Splinting a Toe*

Toes are splinted by taping them to their neighbor. This method allows for self-rescue or trip continuation at the victim's option.

DISLOCATION

A joint is dislocated when one end of a ball joint slips out of its socket, or the bones of a joint become separated. Shoulder and finger dislocations are common injuries that can be repaired by first-aid methods. A finger dislocation can occur when you trip and fall on extended fingers. Often a finger fracture and dislocation occur at the same time.

A typical shoulder dislocation occurs in the sport of kayaking when the paddler's arm is fully extended out and away from the body and the force of the current suddenly rotates the arm backwards. This is a painful injury. Dislocations require that pain medication be given quickly and the dislocation be restored to its normal position as soon as possible. They become more difficult to treat with time due to severe muscle spasm.

☞ *Signs of Finger Dislocation*
- Compared to other fingers, a dislocated finger looks crooked and deformed.
- Swelling and pain accompany the deformity.

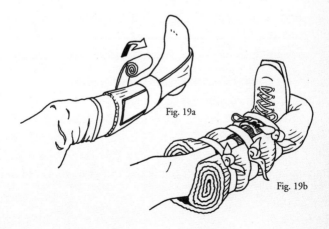

Fig. 19a

Fig. 19b

✢ *Treating a Dislocated Finger*

1. Grasp the base of the finger in one hand and the end of the finger in the other hand. Apply traction with a straight, steady pull until the finger appears straight when compared to the other fingers. (This will not work with the knuckle of the index finger, which requires surgery for realignment.)

2. Insert a 3- or 4-inch square cotton bandage between the fingers for padding. Splint the finger to one or two adjacent fingers with tape.

3. Medicate for pain with ibuprofen. (See **Appendix A** for alternative medications.)

☛ *Signs of Dislocated Shoulder*

Shoulder dislocations occur commonly in people who have had them before. They often can tell you what the diagnosis is and how to fix it.

- Shoulder loses its normal rounded shape.
- The arm is held away from the chest.
- Numbness and/or tingling in hand and arm; pulse in wrist may be weak or absent.
- Arm is weak and victim is reluctant to move it voluntarily.

✢ *Treating a Dislocated Shoulder*

Treat in the field only if evacuation to medical care will require more than 2 hours, or if evacuation would be dangerous for the victim.

1. Have the subject lie down on a flat piece of ground. Support his arm with gentle traction as he moves into position on his back.

2. Apply a gentle, straight pull (traction) to the arm, maintaining a 90-degree angle and a bent elbow (see Fig. 20). A second person to keep the injured person from sliding is helpful.
3. Maintain a gentle, straight pull (traction) while slowly rotating the arm into a baseball pitch position (see Fig. 20).
4. Maintain position until the victim's shoulder muscles fatigue and relax, at which time the shoulder will rotate back into its socket. This can take up to 15 minutes. Stop if pain increases. The dislocation is repaired when the pain dramatically improves and full range of movement in the arm returns.
5. Apply arm sling and binder (see Fig. 16, page 78) and evacuate to definitive medical care.

If reduction is unsuccessful, apply arm sling and binder and evacuate.

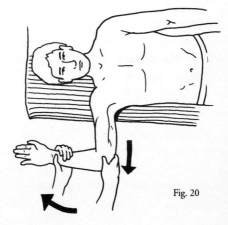

Fig. 20

Altitude Sickness

As altitude increases, the amount of oxygen in the blood decreases. The body's response to a lower concentration of oxygen is to increase the rate of breathing. The illnesses caused by exposure to high altitude occur as a result of the decreased oxygen available to the system. The more severe the oxygen deficit (the difference between what the body requires for normal function, and what is available) and the more rapidly the deficit is forced upon the system (by climbing too high, too fast) the worse the symptoms and potential consequences will be. Additionally, this change in the pattern of breathing increases the amount of water lost through the nose and mouth as we breathe, and also increases the level of work done by the muscles of the rib cage and the diaphragm. To compensate, the body requires more calories and more water.

A body at rest at sea level requires about 2 quarts (liters) of water a day to maintain normal functions. With strenuous activity at altitude, the fluid requirement can easily double or triple. The same ratio applies to the body's caloric needs. It takes about 2,000 calories a day to maintain bodily functions while performing a mild day's work at sea level, but that requirement can double or triple with strenuous activity at altitude. If you climb too quickly for your body to adjust, or without adequate fluid and calorie replacement, you will very likely get sick.

High-altitude edema, or swelling of the ankles, is not associated with serious illness in previously healthy climbers or trekkers and requires no specific treatment. Acute mountain sickness, high-altitude pulmonary edema (known as HAPE—the buildup of abnormal lung fluid) and high-altitude cerebral edema (known as HACE—swelling of the brain) are progressively severe illnesses caused by climbing too high, too fast. The risk for all of these illnesses increases without adequate fluid and calorie intake. HAPE and HACE are potentially fatal illnesses.

Everyone's system adapts to changes in altitude at different rates. Children acclimatize much more slowly than adults and are at greater risk for HAPE and HACE. Young adults adapt more slowly than older adults. While the ability to do work (climb, carry a heavy pack) at high altitude depends on how aerobically fit you are, the likelihood of your suffering altitude sickness does not depend directly on fitness.

Prescription medications can treat the symptoms of altitude sickness, but they are not a substitute for descent. Do not allow a person with the signs of altitude sickness to descend alone.

FIRST-AID TIP:
The increased rate of breathing at altitude can cause a dry, raspy throat. Carry throat lozenges on high-altitude trips.

Preventing Acute Mountain Sickness (AMS)
1. Climb slowly at altitudes above 7,000 feet if you live at or near sea level. Plan for rest days as altitude increases,

and be prepared for unavoidable delays due to slow acclimatization. People acclimate at their own rate. A rough guideline would be: do not sleep more than a thousand feet higher than you did the night before.

2. Don't wait until you are thirsty to begin replacing fluids. Drink water several times an hour. Maintain a clear and plentiful urine.

3. Above 10,000 feet, 70 percent of your calorie intake should come from carbohydrates, with the remaining calories evenly divided between protein and fat sources. Get into the habit of eating small amounts of high carbohydrate food continuously throughout the day.

4. Avoid lack of sleep, fatigue, and hypothermia; they increase both the likelihood of getting ill and the severity of symptoms. Take it slow and easy until you are acclimatized.

☛ *Signs of Acute Mountain Sickness (AMS)*
- Mild to moderately severe headache.
- Loss of appetite.
- Loss of energy, as if you had the flu.
- Nausea, occasional vomiting.
- Difficulty sleeping.
- Low urine output.

✚ *Treating Acute Mountain Sickness (AMS)*
1. Force yourself to drink 4-5 quarts (liters) a day of clear fluid, including soups and drinks.
2. Force yourself to eat; you cannot overeat on a high-altitude climb.

3. Do not climb higher until symptoms disappear.

4. Climb down if the symptoms are not improved in one or two days, immediately if they get worse. A descent of 500–1,000 feet should provide rapid improvement.

5. Treat headache with ibuprofen. (See **Appendix A** for alternative medications.)

6. Treat nausea with a prescription anti-nausea medication such as Compazine. Consult your physician. (See **Appendix A** for alternative medications.)

7. Insomnia and other symptoms of mild altitude sickness can be treated with Diamox, a prescription medication that people allergic to sulfa drugs cannot take. This medication can also prevent the onset of acute mountain sickness for some climbers, if started one day before the climb above 8,000-9,000 feet begins, but cannot safely be substituted for a slow ascent or rapid descent if symptoms persist longer than a day or two. Consult your physician.

☞ *Signs of High-Altitude Pulmonary Edema (HAPE)*
HAPE and High-Altitude Cerebral Edema (HACE) can occur simultaneously. Each is a critical, life-threatening illness. Together they represent a potential catastrophe. Onset of symptoms can be very rapid. If you ignore the symptoms of AMS and continue to climb, you will be at high risk for HAPE or HACE.

- Weakness and fatigue which are much greater than that experienced by other members of the party who are in equally good physical condition.
- Extreme shortness of breath with exertion.

- Dry or raspy cough, often mistaken for bronchitis.
- Breathing rate greater than 20 breaths per minute after 20 minutes of rest.
- Heart rate greater than 130 beats per minute after 20 minutes of rest.
- Blue lips and nailbeds.
- Gurgling sounds in the chest (often misdiagnosed as "pneumonia").
- Symptoms often worse during the night and in the early morning hours.

Severely ill HAPE victims may become confused, irrational or delirious. Assume this is a sign that HACE is also present and that the situation is critical.

✛ *Treating High-Altitude Pulmonary Edema (HAPE)*

1. Immediately descend 2,000-4,000 feet. Do this before the victim becomes so sick she cannot descend under her own power. Descent is the standard treatment for anyone with signs of major altitude illness.
2. Keep the victim warm.
3. Use oxygen on descent, if available (2 liter per minute flow).

Mild symptoms of HAPE can be treated by experienced personnel with Diamox, a prescription medication not suitable for sulfa-drug allergic persons. Consult your physician. More severe symptoms can be treated by experienced personnel with medication that lowers the pressure in the pulmonary blood vessels and with a potent anti-inflammatory medication. None of these medications are a substitute for descent.

☞ *Signs of High-Altitude Cerebral Edema (HACE)*

HAPE and HACE can occur at the same time. Each is a critical life-threatening illness; appearing together, they represent a potential catastrophe. Onset of the symptoms of HACE can be very rapid.

Watch for:

- Loss of balance or frequent stumbling (ataxia).
- Extremely severe headache.
- Confusion, irrationality, and delirium.
- Temporary blindness.
- Hallucinations.
- Coma.

✚ *Treating High-Altitude Cerebral Edema (HACE)*

There is no lifesaving substitute for immediate descent. Oxygen may be used to buy time to make the necessary descent of 2,000–4,000 feet. Dexamethasone, a prescription medication administered by experienced personnel, may also be used to buy time. Consult your physician.

Cold and Exposure Problems

HYPOTHERMIA (LOW BODY TEMPERATURE)

Hypothermia is defined as a drop in temperature below 95 degrees F. This occurs when the body loses its ability to generate enough heat to maintain normal temperature. Hypothermia claims most of its victims at temperatures between 30 and 50 degrees F. Wind, rain, wet clothing, or falling into cold water increase the loss of heat and hasten the onset. Dehydration and inadequate calorie intake also accelerate the drop in body temperature.

You do not need to take someone's temperature in the backcountry to make the diagnosis or provide treatment. In a hospital, temperature is measured rectally—but this is impractical and potentially life-threatening when treating severe hypothermia in the backcountry. Instead, treat symptoms and monitor by paying close attention to the victim's state of alertness, level of comfort, and urine output. If your first-aid kit contains a disposable oral thermometer, use the readings as a rough guide to the actual core temperature (which will usually be about 1 degree higher than the oral reading) and continue to monitor the victim for signs of improvement.

Preventing Hypothermia

The most important element in preventing hypothermia is to remain dry. Controlling the layer of moisture next to your skin with a layered clothing system is the most effective means of doing so.

Lightweight or midweight synthetic tops and bottoms are a sensible first layer in any cold-weather clothing system. Over this layer, top and bottom, wear an ultralight nylon microfiber layer, such as a runner's windshell and windpants. This combination quickly moves moisture away from the skin. The water vapor moves through the first layers and condenses on the outer microfiber layer, keeping the skin dry and warm. Synthetics do not absorb more than 10 percent of their weight in water, and are quicker to dry than wool, which soaks up 30 percent of its weight. Cotton absorbs too much moisture to be effective in a cold-weather system.

The middle layer(s) you choose depends on the air temperature, wind-chill, activity level, and altitude. It should consist of a light, medium, or heavy fleece or wool top and bottom.

Your outer layer is a windproof and waterproof shell.

In order to keep the base layer as dry as possible, adjust your pace to prevent overheating, and strip off middle layers and shell as necessary.

Remember, if your hands and feet feel cold, cover your head, ears, and neck.

Other preventive steps:

- Don't wait until you are thirsty to begin to replace fluids. Drink a pint (500ml) of water before the start of a day's activities. Drink a glassful every 20-30 minutes while exerting yourself. Monitor the adequacy of fluid intake by maintaining a large volume of clear urine.

- Eat small snacks of nutritionally balanced food throughout the day. Carbohydrates and fats are necessary fuels for endurance activities.

☞ *Signs of Mild Hypothermia*

- Person feels cold, and feet and hands feel painfully cold.
- Shivering, the body's attempt to warm itself, begins as temperature drops below 98–97 degrees F.
- Stumbling or loss of balance and coordination appears as the temperature continues to drop.
- Slurred speech is a symptom of increasingly severe hypothermia.

✚ *Treating Mild Hypothermia*

1. Find or build an emergency shelter at the onset of shivering—put up your tent, dig a snow trench, etc.
2. Build a small fire if below timberline.
3. Change into dry clothes.
4. Drink hot, sweet drinks. Avoid coffee or tea, since they induce excess urine output and can worsen dehydration.
5. Get into a sleeping bag, insulated from the ground. Place canteens of hot water wrapped in items of clothing inside sleeping bag, alongside your neck, groin, and armpits.

Persons who recover all faculties and normal temperature do not require evacuation.

☛ *Signs of Severe Hypothermia*

- Temperature drops below 95 degrees F.
- Shivering stops; victim can no longer rewarm herself without assistance.
- Extreme irritability and irrational judgment.
- Victim may not recognize the need to warm herself.
- Severe lack of coordination; victim may not be able to walk or stand without help.
- Level of consciousness severely impaired.
- Victim may appear to be dead (pulse, heartbeat, breathing difficult to detect, pupils fixed and dilated), but treatment and rescue breathing should not be abandoned until the victim's body temperature is normal.

✚ *Treating Severe Hypothermia*

1. Move the victim to shelter gently.
2. Change her into dry clothing. Do this without sudden movements.
3. Follow all of the above measures used to field treat mild hypothermia. Note that rewarming may take more than a day.
4. One or two warm, dry rescuers may get into two sleeping bags zipped together with the victim.
5. Arrange for evacuation by helicopter if possible (see **Getting Help**, pages 27-28).

Note: A cold or frozen person without apparent heartbeat or respiration should receive only rescue breathing; standard CPR chest compression could trigger a fatal cardiac rhythm.

FROSTBITE

Frostbite is a thermal injury caused by freezing of tissues. The ultimate effects of frostbite over time are similar to those of a burn of similar size and depth. Tissue is lost and function is compromised. Prevention and early recognition of frostbite are the best ways to keep fingers and toes.

Preventing Frostbite

1. Allow sufficient room in boots and gloves to avoid blood vessel constriction.
2. Wear a layered clothing system (see page 91). Do not wear cotton clothing next to your skin during cold-weather work and sports. Mittens are warmer than gloves.
3. Maintain hydration with 4-5 quarts (liters) a day of clear fluid, including the water in soups and juice, in addition to snacks. This should maintain a plentiful flow of clear, colorless urine. If it does not, increase your fluid intake. In cold-weather activities, snack continuously throughout the day on nutritionally balanced foods.
4. Avoid excessive sweating; set a cold-weather pace that does not cause overheating.

☞ *Signs of Frostbite*

- Affected tissues (fingers, ears, toes, face, nose) are cold, pale, and painful.
- As depth of freezing progresses, tissue begins to turn white and feel numb. If freezing continues, tissues will become hard and stiff as ice.

✛ *Treating Frostbite*

1. Rewarm affected parts, immersing in water at 100–104 degrees F. Rewarm in a wilderness setting only if the following conditions are met:

   a. The frostbitten extremity can be kept warm on the way out. If there is a risk it will refreeze, do not rewarm since this freeze-rewarm-freeze cycle increases tissue damage.

   b. Adequate shelter and equipment (heat source, fuel, water) are available.

   c. Strong painkillers are available. Rewarming causes considerable pain as the tissue circulation returns. Ibuprofen will control some of the pain and possibly lower the risk of tissue damage from blood clots in the injured tissue. Consult your physician. (See **Appendix A** for alternative medications.)

2. Evacuate without rewarming if these conditions cannot be met (see **Getting Help**, pages 27-28).

Near Drowning

As far as we know, medical interest in reviving people who suffered submersion or near drowning dates back to eighteenth-century England, when a society for research into and treatment of near-drowning victims was founded. A book published in 1774 described the use of mouth-to-mouth breathing on people who appeared to have drowned.

✤ *Treating a Near-Drowning Victim*

1. Assess victim immediately for ABCs (see pages 20-21) and initiate rescue breathing and CPR as quickly as you can.
2. Immobilize the spine in victims of diving accidents (see **Spinal Injury**, pages 44-47).
3. If the victim's chest does not rise and fall with rescue breathing, perform the Heimlich maneuver (pages 29-31) to clear the airway.
4. Assume the victim is hypothermic. Take off her wet clothing and replace with dry clothing; wrap in extra clothes or sleeping bags; and insulate her from ground with sleeping pads, ropes, etc.
5. Continue CPR until professional help is reached or all rescuers are exhausted.
6. Evacuate to a medical facility even if the victim recovers and feels "fine." There are delayed complications of near drowning that require medical care.

Bites and Stings

WILD ANIMAL BITES

All victims of animal bites need to be professionally evaluated due to the risk of contracting rabies. This means you must evacuate all such victims, even those bitten by small animals or rodents. Vaccination must be accomplished as quickly as possible.

✚ Treating Wild Animal Bites

1. Stop all bleeding. In an animal attack, there may be multiple bleeding wounds; treat as other bloody wounds (see pages 48-50). DO NOT close an animal (or human) bite wound.

2. If you are more than one day from professional medical care, start an oral antibiotic from your first-aid kit following instructions on the label. You must know about medical allergies before you give anyone (including yourself) an antibiotic. Consult your physician. (See **Appendix A** for alternative medications.)

SNAKEBITES

According to the medical literature, a typical snakebite victim in the United States is an intoxicated, adolescent male who gets bitten while trying to handle a poisonous snake. Many, if not most, of the small number (less than ten) of snakebite deaths each year occur in this group of adolescent males when they are bitten many hours from medical care. One third of viper bites in North America are "dry"—there is no envenomation. Most envenomations cause extreme pain at the bite site immediately, marked swelling, and severe bruising within 15 minutes.

All accredited United States hospitals stock pit viper antivenin. If you are generally healthy, stay calm and rational, and get to the hospital within several hours, your chances of surviving a poisonous snakebite are virtually 100 percent.

✚ *Treating Snakebites*

1. Keep the victim calm.
2. Clean the area gently with soap or surgical scrub.
3. Bandage lightly with a sterile bandage, 3 or 4 inches square.
4. Splint an upper extremity bite, and keep at or below heart level.
5. Evacuate to a medical facility without delay. Catching and killing the snake is not necessary. Current antivenin covers all North American species of pit vipers, including rattlesnakes, cotton mouths, and copperheads. Victim can walk out if able. Serious symptoms take several hours to appear.

DO NOT make cuts on skin or use tourniquets, pressure dressings, or electrical currents to treat snakebite.

TICK BITES

Ticks are found in dry brushy areas all over the United States; in the West they are found in sagebrush and along creek bottoms, among other places. They sense your presence by smell and jump onto you as you pass. Several illnesses are transmitted to humans by tick bites. All of them, including Lyme disease, can be cured with antibiotics if brought to a physician's attention promptly.

Preventing Tick Bites

During tick season (spring, summer) wear long pants and shirtsleeves. Tuck pants into socks or tape the boot-sock margin with duct tape. This prevents ticks from reaching the darker and more-difficult-to-self-examine groin, genital, and rectal areas. Wearing light-colored clothing makes it easier to find ticks that have jumped onto you.

Low DEET concentration insect repellent (35 percent or less) can be applied to exposed skin; avoid overuse, especially in young children. (Extremely high concentration DEET has been noted to induce cancers in mice.)

After a day outdoors in spring and summer, examine yourself and your children for ticks. Be sure to search hair, groin, and rectal areas, and look between toes and under arms. If you find a tick, don't panic. Ticks take several hours to attach themselves, and 24-48 hours to transmit disease-causing agents carried in their saliva to humans.

✚ *Removing a Tick*

Carry a needle-nosed forceps in your first-aid kit to remove the tick if it is embedded in your skin.

1. Grasp the tick close to the embedded head.
2. Pull gently in a straight back motion. Do not twist. If the entire tick is removed a small piece of your skin will usually come off with it. Avoid crushing the tick and contaminating your skin with tick blood and body fluids.

3. Scrub the area with soap and water or surgical scrub, and cover with a one-inch plastic bandage. Then wash your hands.
4. Disinfect your forceps after use by boiling.

✚ *Treating Tick Bites*

If you get sick after a tick bite or develop a rash of any kind, consult your doctor. The serious illnesses caused by tick bites, including Lyme disease, can be treated successfully in the early stages—the earlier the better.

INSECT BITES AND STINGS

Stings from bees, wasps, and yellowjackets are most common in North America. In the southeastern and parts of the southwestern United States, fire ant bites can cause a severe, life-threatening allergic reaction. About 1 percent of people are at risk for severe (anaphylactic) reaction from insect bites and stings. There are more fatalities in the United States each year from insect stings than from snakebites.

✚ *Treating Insect Bites and Stings*

1. Wash bite site with soap and water or surgical scrub.
2. Remove stinger if you can see it protruding from bite site. Use a needle-nosed forceps from your first-aid kit. You can also use a commercial venom extractor to extract the venom or insect stinger; follow instructions on extractor kit.
3. Apply a commercial after-bite wipe or low-concentration cortisone cream.
4. To prevent infection, cover bite with an elastic bandage.
5. Use non-prescription antihistamines (such as Benadryl)

to reduce itching and discomfort. (See **Appendix A** for alternative medications.)

SEVERE ALLERGIC (ANAPHYLACTIC) REACTIONS

Severe allergic reactions can occur as a result of insect bites or medication allergy. Such reactions can progress to respiratory and cardiac arrest. Wilderness trekkers with a history of severe allergic reactions are advised to consult their physician regarding the appropriate use of an insect sting kit that contains two powerful, potentially lifesaving medications, epinephrine and diphenhydramine.

☛ *Signs of Severe Allergic (Anaphylactic) Reaction*

- Rapid onset of severe itching, hives, and swelling around the bite.
- Severe swelling around lips, mouth, tongue, or throat, and difficulty swallowing.
- Rapid onset of difficulty in breathing; wheezing and chest tightness.

✛ *Treating Severe Allergic (Anaphylactic) Reaction*

1. Follow the instructions on your prescription anaphylactic reaction kit (Ana-sting or Epi-Pen come with preloaded syringes of epinephrine for self injection).
2. Be prepared to provide immediate **CPR** (pages 18-25).
3. Use non-prescription antihistamines (diphenhydramine and others) to reduce itching and swelling and to prevent recurrence of anaphylaxis symptoms.
4. Evacuate for prompt medical attention. Self-evacuation is OK if the person feels well enough to travel. Be prepared to re-administer the sting-kit medications if symptoms recur.

Eye Conditions

Warning signs of a vision-threatening condition are the appearance of severe pain in the eye or diminished vision. All vision-threatening eye conditions require rapid evacuation. Self-evacuation is OK. Patch the eye for comfort (see page 105) and seek immediate medical attention.

RED EYE AND SNOW BLINDNESS

Most common viral and bacterial infections, irritations, snow blindness, and allergic reactions appear as red eye (conjunctivitis) on examination. This refers to the appearance of the conjunctiva—the membrane that covers the white part of the eye and lines the eyelid. The most commonly occurring causes of red eye are not a threat to vision.

Preventing Snow Blindness

Eyes that are unprotected in strong sun, especially in the snow or on glaciers at high altitude, or on water or reflective sand, can get sunburned. Preventive measures include the use of sunglasses that block 100 percent of ultraviolet light and at least 90 percent of visible light.

☛ *Signs of Red Eye (Conjunctivitis)*
- White of the eye appears bright pink or red; lifting the upper lid exposes abnormally red, inflamed tissue.
- Itching, burning, tearing, yellowish or greenish discharge, crusted eyelashes.

- Vision is not disturbed except possibly mild blurring caused by increased tearing or sticky mucous discharge.
- The eye moves in all directions without paralysis or pain, although movement may increase tearing and make it feel as if something is in the eye.

✢ Treating Red Eye (Conjunctivitis) and Snow Blindness

1. Irrigate material draining from the eye with clean water. Repeat irrigation as often as necessary to clear material draining from the eye.
2. Definitive treatment requires 2 drops of antibiotic eye drops in the eye every 2 hours while person is awake. Garamycin Sulfate is recommended. Consult your physician if you wish to carry this medication in your backcountry first aid kit. Do this for no more than 3 days. DO NOT patch the eye.
3. If conjunctivitis persists for more than 3 days, evacuate victim to a medical facility.

OBJECT IN THE EYE

A small foreign body may be seen easily if it is on the white part of the eye, and seen with more difficulty if lodged in the clear portion of the eye—the cornea. Use a flashlight to examine the clear part of the eye; by moving the beam of light around, you may see the foreign body. If you do not see a foreign body, retract the upper eyelid over a cotton-tipped applicator stick (see Figs. 21a-b, page 104) and look for it on the inside of the upper eyelid.

✤ *Treating Object in the Eye*

1. Touch the tip of a moistened cotton-tipped applicator gently to the object. It should come away on the cotton. If it doesn't come away on the tip of the applicator, irrigate the eye gently with clean water. Have the person lie down on her side, direct the stream of water into the outside corner of the eye, and allow the water to run down across the eye. Have the person blink rapidly while you do this.

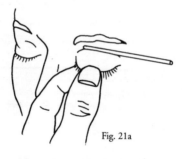

Fig. 21a

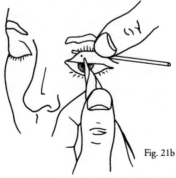

Fig. 21b

2. If the object (such as a sliver of metal, rock, or fish hook) has penetrated either the white or the clear part of the eye, patch the eye and evacuate quickly to a medical facility. Self-evacuation is OK and pain medication may be necessary. *People with an eye patch should not travel out alone.* Their depth perception is impaired and they will not be able to navigate steep or rocky trails without help.

✚ Patching the Eye

DO NOT patch red eyes that are draining a mucousy or pus-like discharge.

1. Have the person close her eye. Place several cotton balls over the lid, and place an eye patch over the cotton balls.
2. Secure the patch in place by taping to the forehead, the cheek, and the nose. No light should enter the patch, and the person should not require any effort to keep her eyelid closed.

Respiratory Infections

EAR, NOSE, AND THROAT INFECTIONS

Ear, nose, and throat infections in adults are most often viral infections, and usually do not require antibiotics in the doctor's office. They are treated with simple, over-the-counter medications that relieve symptoms. If you are in the backcountry for an extended stay, you may want to consult a physician and carry prescription antibiotics because this group of disorders can linger on, and develop a secondary bacterial infection, which requires antibiotic treatment.

☛ *Signs of an Ear, Nose, or Throat Infection*
- Mild headache, low-grade fever, sore throat, ear pain, and sinus pain, with or without drainage from the nose or throat.
- Otherwise healthy adult or adolescent.

✚ *Treatment of an Ear, Nose, or Throat Infection*
1. Maintain hydration with abundant clear fluids.
2. Use one of the over-the-counter nasal sprays for nasal decongestion. Follow instructions on the label.
3. Consult a physician if you would like the option of treating yourself with an antibiotic.

BRONCHITIS AND PNEUMONIA

Pneumonia starts in the air passages (bronchi), but progresses to infect the lung tissue itself. The symptoms of bronchitis and pneumonia are similar and, in the field, they are treated much the same. Bronchitis can be disabling in recreationists with asthma, smokers, or persons with other chronic lung diseases, all of whom are more prone to infection. If treatment does not produce real improvement in two or three days, evacuate.

☛ *Signs of Bronchitis and Pneumonia*

- Persistent, irritating cough that becomes productive of thick, green or yellow mucous, usually after a cold or upper respiratory infection. Pneumonia can occur without a cold first.
- Low-grade fever (less than 101 degrees F) possible. Higher fever (102 degrees F or more) may indicate more severe infection and requires prompt medical attention.
- Mild fatigue common, but extreme fatigue, dry nonproductive cough, and shortness of breath should be interpreted as indicating a more severe condition requiring evacuation, especially if at altitude above eight thousand feet.

✚ *Treating Bronchitis and Pneumonia*

1. Maintain hydration with oral fluids.
2. Consult a physician if you feel you would like the option of treating yourself with an antibiotic.

Abdominal Pain

The most common causes of abdominal pain in the backcountry are food- and water-caused "poisoning" (gastroenteritis) of viral, bacterial, or parasitic (*Giardia*) origin; indigestion from a change in diet; and constipation. Diarrheal illness—bowel movements that are watery and have no shape of their own—is caused by bacteria or virus ingested with food or water. Diarrhea can occur anywhere, but you are most at risk if you drink untreated water or eat raw fruits and vegetables in underdeveloped parts of the world.

The most important thing to learn is how to recognize serious abdominal pain, which can be life threatening and requires immediate evacuation to a medical facility.

☞ *Signs of Serious Abdominal Pain Requiring Emergency Evacuation*

Each of the following symptoms, alone or in combination, signifies a condition that may require surgery, and victims must be immediately evacuated:

- Moderate to severe pain that comes with nausea and vomiting, or vomiting blood.
- Pain that lasts for more than 6 hours.
- Pain that prevents sleep.
- Pain with abdomen appearing bloated or distended.
- Pain localized to a single point or portion of the abdomen, not generalized over the entire abdomen.
- A rigid, boardlike abdomen.

✤ *Treating Serious Abdominal Pain*

1. People with serious abdominal emergencies are rarely, if ever, able to self-evacuate. Getting help with their evacuation and rescue will almost always be necessary. Do not leave the victim alone, and if possible, send two people for help (see **Getting Help**, pages 27-28).
2. Do not give fluids.
3. Try not to move the victim.

CONSTIPATION

Constipation is common on wilderness trips, given the change in diet and environment from what we are accustomed to. Many people have daily bowel movements at home and, for them, a period of 3 to 5 days without a bowel movement is defined as constipation. Bowel movements are so variable from one person to another, however, that constipation may also be defined as a delay in bowel movement that makes a person uncomfortable.

Constipation is best prevented by increasing the fiber, fruits, and liquids in your diet. On a wilderness adventure, beans, prunes, and dehydrated apricots are excellent sources of fiber and provide a means of managing constipation "naturally."

Over-the-counter laxatives such as Senokot, Ducolax, and others are safe for occasional use, but avoid using them more often than every 5 to 7 days.

TRAVELERS DIARRHEA

Travelers Diarrhea often appears in several trip companions at about the same time, which is a hint that its origin is in food or water. Gastroenteritis and appendicitis can, in the early stages, present themselves in a similar fashion—but diarrhea in appendicitis is rare. Pain in appendicitis is localized, usually to the right side of the abdomen.

Preventing Food- or Water-Caused Illness

1. Boil, filter, or chemically treat all water in the backcountry (see **Water Purification**, pages 113-115).
2. Do not drink tapwater or use ice cubes in underdeveloped areas of the world. Bottled and carbonated water or drinks usually are safe to drink in undeveloped countries.
3. If traveling in underdeveloped countries, do not eat fruits or vegetables you have not peeled. Avoid salads, salsa, reheated foods, milk, and milk products.
4. Take bismuth salicylates in tablets (such as Pepto-Bismol) or liquid form to prevent Travelers Diarrhea in high risk areas. **Note:** People with an allergy to aspirin cannot take this medication. Using salicylates at the recommended dosages can cause stomach bleeding.

☞ *Signs of Travelers Diarrhea (Gastroenteritis)*

- Mild, widespread abdominal pain that starts gradually and builds in intensity. Pain comes in waves or cramps— usually between cramps the abdomen is pain-free, or very nearly so.
- Nausea and vomiting, up to 10-20 times a day.
- Moderately severe, watery diarrhea, up to 10-20 times a day.
- Symptoms often appear within the first 2-3 days of a visit to an underdeveloped area.
- Low-grade fever (less than 101 degrees F) possible.

✚ *Treating Travelers Diarrhea (Gastroenteritis)*

Gastroenteritis symptoms that persist for more than three days, treated or untreated, require evacuation to a medical facility. Self-rescue is OK if diarrhea is the main symptom.

1. Replace fluid loss from vomiting and diarrhea—this is critical. Use fruit juice (bottled if traveling in an under-developed area), broth, soup, or sports drinks plus oral replacement salts. About 1 quart of fluids an hour may be required in the first 8 hours.

2. Carry oral rehydration salts on trips to areas where Travelers Diarrhea is common. Mix with treated water to make 1 quart of balanced replacement fluid per package.

3. Treat mild nausea accompanying gastroenteritis with prescription medications such as Compazine, if desired. Consult your physician. Persons with severe nausea and vomiting should be evacuated. (See **Appendix A** for alternative medications.)

4. Loperamide, an anti-diarrheal, or bismuth salicylate (Pepto-Bismol) tablets may be purchased over-the-counter to slow down the diarrhea. Follow the instructions on the label. DO NOT use if there is blood or pus in the diarrhea. Persons allergic to aspirin should not use salicylates, since even recommended dosages can cause stomach bleeding.

5. An oral antibiotic, Ciprofloxin, can shorten the duration of Travelers Diarrhea by several days. Consult your physician. (See **Appendix A** for alternative medications.)

GIARDIA

Giardia is a parasitic protozoan that lives in fresh water contaminated with animal or human fecal matter. While it may be present anywhere, including the water supply of many big cities, it requires quite a few *Giardia* to make you sick. *Giardia* causes a chronic form of diarrhea and abdominal pain, both of which are much less severe than the acute condition caused by waterborne bacteria and viruses. The symptoms of *Giardia* typically appear a week to ten days after exposure, which is much longer than the immediate onset of bacterial Travelers Diarrhea. To prevent *Giardia* infection, see **Water Purification**, pages 113-115.

☞ *Signs of Giardia*

Most people have no symptoms with *Giardia* infection—or only mild, widespread, abdominal bloating and discomfort, which usually begins 7-10 days after ingestion of *Giardia*-contaminated water. Accurate diagnosis requires examination and laboratory workup. Some symptoms are:

- Burps and flatus that smell like "rotten eggs."
- Bowel movements 3-4 times a day, producing stools that are soft, bulky, and foul smelling.
- Loss of appetite or mild nausea.

✤ *Treating Giardia*

Most *Giardia*-infected people recover in a week or two, without treatment; they develop an immunity to the parasite. Metronidazole, an oral antibiotic, is a standard medical treatment for *Giardia*.

Consult your physician once out of the backcountry if symptoms persist.

Water Purification

Contaminated surface water is a fact of life in the modern wilderness. Long gone are the days when a refreshing drink of water could be sipped from every stream along the trail, let alone wells or taps at campgrounds and recreation areas. Bacteria, parasites, and viruses are carried from watershed to watershed in the feces of domestic cattle, wildlife, and people. They have turned a simple drink of crystal-clear water into a risky game of chance.

In North America and Europe, the list of common waterborne microorganisms that cause human illness is long and, unfortunately, growing. Major culprits in 1997 are *E. coli, Giardia,* Hepatitis A, *Salmonella,* and *Campylobacter.* In the underdeveloped world, disease-causing viruses, including those that induce Hepatitis B (a potentially fatal illness), inhabit most surface and tap water. Cold water is no protection against infection, since it actually prolongs the lifespan of most microorganisms, and freezing simply puts them to sleep until the spring melt.

Three methods of disinfecting water are discussed below, and each has strengths and weaknesses. Choose a convenient primary method of disinfection depending upon your destination, equipment, and preference, and have a backup method as insurance.

Boiling

Boiling water kills all living organisms known to cause human illness. Regardless of the altitude, by the time water boils it is safe to drink—the temperature required to kill any of the organisms that cause waterborne illness, viruses included, is reached long before the boiling point. Heating water to disinfect it is virtually foolproof, but requires a stove, abundant fuel, and a pot. That makes boiling an ideal purification method for winter trips where your water will come from ice and snow that has to be melted anyway, and less convenient if you are traveling light, touring and trekking from guest house to guest house in rural Asia, in which case iodine tablets might be better.

Pouring boiled water back and forth between containers as it cools aerates the water and improves the taste, as does mixing it with a powdered lemonade or sport drink.

Chemical Treatment

Iodine tablets, sold under the trade names of Potable Aqua and Globaline, will kill all bacteria, parasites, and viruses found in surface water or tap water. That makes iodine water purification a good choice for traveling light, trekking, biking, or hosteling across remote territory. Iodine's killing power, however, is time- and temperature-dependent. The colder and more cloudy the water, the more iodine tablets are required to disinfect it, and the longer it takes.

Allow cloudy water to settle, then pour off the top layer to reduce the amount of organic and inorganic matter available to interfere with the action of the iodine. Iodine taste can be masked with powdered lemonade or sport drink.

Follow these guidelines:

- Cold, clear, high-altitude creek water far from human habitation and domestic livestock requires one iodine tablet dissolved in 1 quart (liter) of water for 30 minutes before it is safe to drink.
- Cold, cloudy water requires two tablets dissolved in a quart (liter) of water for 30-45 minutes before it is safe to drink.
- Warm, clear water requires one tablet dissolved in a quart of water for 10 minutes.
- Warm, cloudy water requires two tablets dissolved in a quart of water for 10 minutes.

Water Purifiers

Water filters are convenient and efficient for warm-weather trips, and most will remove parasites, cysts, and bacteria that cause human waterborne illness. On the other hand, they freeze up in cold weather and require frequent cleaning or replacement of the filtration element. They cannot be counted on to kill all viruses that contaminate drinking water. Several companies sell water purifiers. These instruments not only filter water, but chemically treat it as well, usually with iodine. They are excellent choices on backpacking, fishing, climbing, rafting, and paddle trips in North America and Europe. In fact, a water purifier (with iodine tablets carried as backup) is a safe and sensible system for just about anywhere.

Vaccinations

Vaccination requirements for foreign travel change frequently. The federal Centers for Disease Control (CDC) in Atlanta, Georgia, is the world's leading center for research and treatment of contagious diseases. The CDC provides up-to-date information on vaccination requirements and malaria prevention for travel to all areas of the world. Call (404) 332-4559 to reach the agency's switchboard.

Current Vaccination Recommendations (1997)

- Tetanus/diphtheria vaccination every ten years.
- Polio booster before traveling in underdeveloped countries.
- Oral typhoid vaccination before traveling in underdeveloped countries.
- Measles vaccination and German measles booster for everyone born after 1956.
- Yellow fever vaccination, with booster every ten years. These shots are required by a number of countries in Central America, South America, and Africa. Consult the CDC for specifics.
- Hepatitis A vaccine is now available. Vaccination is recommended for backcountry travel in underdeveloped countries.
- Hepatitis B vaccine is recommended for backcountry stays in underdeveloped countries where contact with blood or semen is likely (especially for medical personnel, emergency personnel, and journalists exposed to violence or victims of violence).

Appendix A

A WILDERNESS FIRST-AID KIT

Ideally, each person or party builds or buys a first-aid kit customized to suit particular needs—based on party size, length of stay in the wilderness, likelihood of professional rescue as opposed to self-rescue, pre-existing medical conditions and allergies, and the specific environmental demands of the trip. An overnight stay 5 miles from the trailhead in the Adirondacks of northern New York in July can present different first-aid challenges than a week-long float down the Middle Fork of the Salmon River in Idaho. A kit that covered a small party on either of these short excursions would be quite different than what is required for a party of four on a month-long Alaskan mountaineering expedition.

The list below is a good place to start. Larger kits and customized options are commercially available from a number of outdoor specialty shops, but resist the temptation to bring more equipment than you feel comfortable using. After you have completed courses in first aid, wilderness first response, and CPR, you will be better able to judge what kit and components are right for you.

BANDAGES AND SURGICAL SUPPLIES

Tape, Adhesive—Use to secure splints, tape down bandages over lacerations and abrasions, etc. Some folks are allergic to the adhesive and are more comfortable with surgical paper tape.

Basic Blister Dressing—Transparent, sterile film dressing such as Tegaderm for covering shallow blisters; permeable to water vapor and oxygen, impermeable to microbes. Apply to dry skin and cover with molefoam and tape. Change if soiled.

Spenco Second Skin—Hydrocolloid dressing used to cover burns; protects wound from contamination, provides rapid pain relief.

Surgical Soap—Non-iodine, non-phenol based mild surgical soap will clean debris and contaminants from the wound surface and will not injure tissue.

Sterile Non-Stick Bandage—4x4-inch; applied directly to cover a clean laceration or abrasion wound surface after it has been cleaned and the wound edges brought together with adhesive strips, sutured, or stapled. Makes dressing changes painless. Apply directly to wound and place 1 or 2 sterile 4x4s on top, then tape in place.

Sterile Bandage—3x3- or 4x4-inch; apply over non-adhering bandage for covering lacerations, abrasions, and open wounds; use as pressure dressing on uncontrolled bleeding of smaller wounds; use as a sterile wipe to pat dry wounds after irrigation, before dressing. (Be sure to wear your vinyl or surgical gloves when cleaning blood or other bodily secretions from skin or elsewhere.)

Cotton Balls—Use for gently cleaning and wiping away dirt, grime, blood, and other secretions on skin, where sterile technique is not required.

Iodine Wipes—Individually packaged. Use to clean skin around wound; do not apply to interior of wound.

Vinyl Gloves—Wear these in any wound care or emergency situation where you may come into contact with bodily fluids, for protection of both the victim and yourself. Latex gloves have caused fatal allergic reactions in unsuspecting victims and are not recommended for backcountry use.

Sterile Applicators—Useful for applying and spreading topical burn wound medication; also useful for ear wax removal, for removal of foreign body on the white part of the eye, and for examining the inside of the upper lid by gently rolling it over the stick. **Note:** These are *not* the commercial cotton swabs generally available in supermarkets and drug stores. Commercial cotton swabs are not sterilized.

Roller Gauze—3-inch-wide, flexible, stretchy gauze; use it to wrap a wound and keep sterile pads in place. Also provides cushioning and protection for the injury.

Plastic Bandage Strips—1-inch wide; for covering minor cuts, scrapes, insect bites, and blisters.

Sunscreen—SPF 15 at least; more at high altitude.

Insect Sting Stick—Apply to insect bites or stings for relief of discomfort.

Flexible Splinting (SAM splint™)—Moldable aluminum splint covered with closed cell foam, marketed under the trade name SAM splint™. Can be cut to size and shape as needed for use on wrist, arm, elbow, or ankle. The splinting is best cut with the kind of all-purpose shears paramedics carry.

Wound Closure Strips—Use to bring together the skin edges of minor cuts.

Eye Pads—To cover an injured, painful, sunblind, or red eye to provide comfort and protection. Do not patch an infected, draining eye.

Tongue Depressors—Use to examine a mouth, throat, or tongue condition, or as small splints for finger injuries; also useful for applying ointments to a large area or as tinder for an emergency fire.

Molefoam—Pressure point padding, often used in conjunction with adhesive or duct tape to prevent blisters in known pressure points. Molefoam is a padded (and more comfortable) version of another blister-preventative product called moleskin.

Duct Tape—Use for fashioning splints, preventing hot spots on feet, immobilizing the neck and spine, and other uses. Wrap about 10 feet of tape around your toothbrush or ski pole to save space.

Cyanoacrylate Glue (SuperGlue)—Use for closing those small, clean, but hard-to-bandage nicks, scrapes, and cuts on fingers, knuckles, and hands that seem to stay open forever. To seal such a wound, pinch and hold the wound edges together, then spread a small dab of glue along the line of injury. Do not apply to the interior of the wound.

SPECIALIZED MEDICAL INSTRUMENTS

Wound Irrigation Syringe—30 ml recommended, with an 18- or 19-gauge hypodermic needle to provide adequate pressure for washing dirt, debris, and microbes from the wound. Also used to clean infectious debris from an infected wound.

Anaphylaxis Emergency Kit—Commercially available by prescription only; follow the instructions on the kit exactly. Use only for life-threatening allergic reactions when prescribed for a victim with a history of severe allergic reactions to medication or insect bite.

Venom Extractor—Suction device, applied directly to wound. These instruments are useful for removing wasp and bee stingers. Some authorities recommend venom extractors for the removal of snakebite venom, but the effectiveness has not been convincingly demonstrated in a practical emergency setting.

Forceps—4.5-inch; use for removing foreign bodies such as splinters, bee stingers, cactus spines, etc. Do not use in removing foreign bodies from the eye.

Scissors—4.5-inch; use to trim or cut off bandages, splints, or scalp hair around a scalp wound before treatment.

Airway Kit—Assorted sizes, child and adult; use to maintain an open upper airway when you perform CPR or rescue breathing.

Survival ("Space") Blanket—Thin, extremely lightweight reflective blanket used to conserve body heat.

NON-PRESCRIPTION MEDICATIONS

Hydrocortisone Cream—1 percent strength; apply a small amount to insect bites, stings, poison ivy, or poison oak skin rashes three or four times a day.

Decongestant Nasal Spray—For colds, stuffy nose, and blocked sinuses of any cause. Two squirts in each nostril, wait five minutes and spray one more time on both sides. Repeat once more during the day.

Bismuth Salicylate Tablets (Pepto-Bismol)—Antidiarrheal, anti-indigestion medication; also recommended for prevention of Travelers Diarrhea in high-risk areas of the world. Not for persons allergic or sensitive to aspirin. Can irritate stomach if overused.

Diphenhydramine—25 mg tablets; antihistamine for symptoms of allergy; also used as sleep medication, but leaves some people with a hung-over feeling the next morning; try it at home first.

Pain Medication—Aspirin, acetaminophen (Tylenol), and ibuprofen each provide the same amount of pain relief. Take 1 to 2 tablets, 3 to 4 times a day. Stomach irritation common with aspirin and ibuprofen.

PRESCRIPTION MEDICATIONS
(CONSULT YOUR PHYSICIAN)

Lorazepam 0.5 mg—A sedative useful for treating acute stress reactions. Can be habit forming. Not for use at high altitude because it slows respiration.

PAIN MEDICATION

Acetaminophen (Tylenol) with Codeine—Oral pain relief equivalent to injectable morphine, with the same risks: depressed respiration at high altitude, daytime drowsiness, nausea, or vomiting. Can be habit forming.

ORAL ANTIBIOTICS

Cephalexin (Keflex)—Used to treat skin and wound infections, and for open fractures if evacuation is delayed.

Trimethoprim/Sulfamethoxazole—Useful for treatment of upper respiratory infection, bladder or urinary tract infection, and as an alternative treatment for Travelers Diarrhea.

Erythromycin (various forms)—Used in place of Penicillin or Cephalexin in Penicillin-allergic people.

ANTINAUSEA MEDICATIONS

Hydroxyzine (Atarax)—Antihistamine that reduces nausea and vomiting due to motion sickness, acute mountain sickness, and other causes. Side effect of daytime drowsiness.

Compazine—The low-dose form of this medication reduces or eliminates nausea in a number of medical conditions; it is safe to use at high altitude, and can be used for a few days as a sleep medication.

Appendix B

To be effective, emergency medical treatment requires accurate and complete information about the victim. The scene of emergency treatment, however, can often be hectic, stressful, and confused. After you've administered first aid, fill out this form and give it to emergency medical personnel.

Victim's name _____

Accident location _____

Time of accident _____

Description of accident and victim's condition immediately following

_____

_____

_____

_____

_____

_____

What was done for victim at accident scene? _____

_____

_____

_____

_____

Appendix C

MEDICAL HISTORY

A thorough medical history of the victim is of inestimable value to doctors in the case of an emergency. To ensure that medical personnel have access to your personal information, carry a completed copy of this form on your person when you travel in the backcountry.

Date _____

Name _____

Address _____

Home telephone _____ Emergency contact _____

Date of birth _____ Height _____ Weight _____

Blood pressure _____ Pulse rate (average) _____

I rate my overall health status as:

poor_____ fair_____ good_____ excellent_____

I rate my current physical condition as:

poor_____ fair_____ good_____ excellent_____

I smoke/do not smoke cigarettes, at the rate of _____ packs/day

Allergies to medications, insect bites, or foods: _____

_____

_____

_____

Medications taken, including all current and recent prescriptions:

_____

_____

_____

Past medical history

I have been afflicted with the following (circled):

Acute mountain sickness	Other heart or lung disease
Heat stroke	_____
Sun/snow blindness	
Frostbite	_____
Hypothermia	Malaria
Bronchitis	Diabetes
Asthma	Epilepsy
Pneumonia	Anemia
Pleurisy	Ulcer Disease
Tuberculosis	Other chronic illness
Rheumatic fever	_____
Heart attack	_____

Past surgical procedures (including complications, if any):

_____

_____

Chronic medical conditions currently suffered: _____

_____

_____

Immunization record

VACCINE	DATE OF MOST RECENT VACCINATION	VACCINE	DATE OF MOST RECENT VACCINATION
Tetanus booster	_____	MMR	_____
Diptheria	_____	Typhoid	_____
Polio	_____		

Current medical condition

I currently am subject to the following (circled):

Head
  Headaches
  Dizzy spells
  Fainting spells
Eyes
  Pain
  Inflammation
  Double vision
  Vision loss
Nose
  Frequent colds
  Chronic sinus trouble
  Postnasal drip
  Nose bleeds
Ears
  Pain
  Discharge
  Ringing
  Hearing loss
Mouth
  Pain
  Bleeding
  Soreness
  Abscessed teeth
Neck
  Pain
  Swelling
  Stiffness
Heart and lungs
  Chest pain
  Palpitations
  Shortness of breath
  Chronic cough

Gastrointestinal
  Abdominal pain
  Nausea
  Vomiting
  Indigestion
  Diarrhea
  Appetite loss
  Constipation
  Bloody, black, or tarry stools
  Clay-colored stools
  Jaundice
  Hemorrhoids
Genitourinary
  Pain during urination
  Increased or decreased frequency of
    urination
  Passage of blood, gravel, or stones
  Menstrual abnormalities
  Cramps
  Excessive menstrual bleeding
Musculoskeletal
  Back pain
  Joint pain
  Muscle cramps
  Weakness
  Paralysis
Skin
  Recurrent rash, abscess, or boils
General
  Fever
  Chills
  Weakness
  Lethargy
  Sleep problems
  Unexplained weight loss

Other information not included: _____

_____

_____

_____

_____

_____

_____

_____

_____

_____

_____

_____

_____

_____